Modern medicine

Modern medicine

Lay perspectives and experiences

Edited by

Simon J. Williams
University of Warwick

Michael Calnan
University of Kent

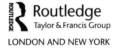

Routledge
Taylor & Francis Group

LONDON AND NEW YORK

© Simon J. Williams, Michael Calnan and contributors 1996

This book is copyright under the Berne Convention.
No reproduction without permission.
All rights reserved.

First published in 1996 by UCL Press

Reprinted 2003 by Routledge
11 New Fetter Lane
London, EC4P 4EE

Routledge is an imprint of the
Taylor & Francis Group

British Library Cataloguing in Publication Data
A catalogue record for this book is available from the British Library.

Library of Congress Cataloguing in Publication Data are available.

ISBNs:
1-85728-317-1 HB
1-85728-318-X PB

Typeset in Palatino.
Printed and Bound by Antony Rowe Ltd

To the memory of Oscar

Contents

CONTENTS

Preface

In contrast to the burgeoning field of research on lay concepts of health and illness, little work has been conducted to date by medical sociologists on lay perspectives, experiences and evaluations of modern medicine and medical care. This is surprising as, notwithstanding the importance of these issues for a range of "medical" and policy-related concerns including patient "compliance", medical "outcomes" and consumer "satisfaction" with health care, research of this nature has crucial implications for the sociological understanding of lay knowledge and experience, as well as some of the more macro-focused theoretical debates surrounding modern medicine and the lay populace in contemporary Western society.

Certainly it is clear that a number of critical changes are occurring in "late" modernity, changes that carry important implications for our understanding of the place and function of modern Western medicine, the future of professional power and dominance, and the role of the lay populace as "consumers" of health care. Here, a number of key developments suggest themselves including: the increasingly technologized nature of modern medicine in which access to the human body is becoming mediated through a vast array of electronic images and digitalized forms of coding (i.e. "virtual" medicine, "hyperreal" bodies); the increasing fragmentation of modern medical knowledge and practice and the transformation of the traditional biomedical paradigm (i.e. "reflexive" or "postmodern" medicine); the role of the mass media in contemporary society as carriers and amplifiers of a more "challenging" position with respect to modern medicine (i.e. the "mediation" of contemporary experience); and finally, the growth of an increasingly informed and reflexive lay populace as knowledge becomes pluralized, systems of authority and expertise "contested", and "alternative" forms of health and healing sought (i.e. "lay re-skilling"). These developments, in turn, have been reinforced through a number of recent policy documents that emphasize "consumer choice", "patient charters", "satisfaction" with health care, "community participation", and the role of "local voices" in health care purchasing.

In short, this suggests a critical and dynamic picture involving elements of "trust" and "doubt" that casts a long shadow over many of the traditional theoretical assumptions concerning the relationship between modern medicine and the lay populace. As such, there is an urgent need not only for further empirical investigation of these issues, but also for the elaboration of new theoretical perspectives in order to capture more accurately this changing and dynamic social landscape.

It is in this context that the rationale for the present volume emerges. In particular, we have sought to bring together, within the scope of a single edited volume, a range of detailed qualitative and ethnographic research from established scholars within the field of medical sociology, concerning lay peoples' own perspectives and experiences of modern medical care and technology. In doing so, the volume as a whole seeks to address, through detailed empirical data, the following key questions. First, how do lay people view modern medicine and what are the nature of their experiences of medical care and technology? Second, what criteria do lay people draw upon in evaluating different forms of medical care and technology? Finally, what, at a theoretical level, does this tell us about the relationship between modern medicine and the lay populace in the contemporary era? Are people, for example, simply passive and accepting, active and critical, or a mixture of both, and to what extent do views on the relative merits of modern medicine differ within different segments of the lay populace?

In addressing these key issues, we hope that the volume as whole will shed further empirical light upon the nature of lay perspectives and experiences of modern medicine, and in doing so, serve to "ground" some of the more abstract theoretical debates surrounding the changing relationship between modern medicine and the lay populace in late twentieth-century western society. Indeed, it is this dialectical interplay between theory and data that lies at the heart of this book.

As with any book venture, it is important to say a few "thank you's". First, we would like to thank Justin Vaughan and UCL Press for helping this book become a reality. Second, thanks go to all the contributors who, not withstanding a few "un-met deadlines", made our editorial task a surprisingly pleasant and largely unproblematic one.

Finally, I (SJW) would also like to say a few personal thank you's: first, to Gill Bendelow, who effectively served as a "ghost editor" throughout the book's gestation and helped keep the project "on the rails" at various crucial stages; secondly, to my parents Betty and Alan Williams for their continual support and encouragement and to Tessa Watkinson for putting up with me more generally; and finally to Viv and Mario for some wonderful meals! Needless to say, any errors in the editing process lie entirely with us.

Simon J. Williams & Michael Calnan,
April 1995

Notes on contributors

Gillian A. Bendelow has recently taken up a lectureship in applied social studies at the University of Warwick. Prior to that she was a research associate at the Social Science Research Unit, Institute of Education, University of London, where she completed her doctoral research. Her current research interests and writing concern the sociology of the body, with particular reference to gender, pain and emotions, and children's health.

Nicky Britten is a lecturer in medical sociology based in the Department of General Practice at the United Medical and Dental Schools of Guy's and St Thomas's Hospitals. Her research interests and publications include the social aspects of drugs and medicines, prescribing, pharmacy and medicine taking.

Michael Bury is Director of Medical Sociology, and Professor of Sociology at Royal Holloway, University of London. He is also responsible for the MSc in medical sociology at Royal Holloway. He has published widely in the areas of ageing, chronic illness, patient views of health care and cultural aspects of medicine, including the impact of the media. He is co-editor of the Journal *Sociology of Health and Illness*. Recent research projects include a national study of quality of life among the very old, social aspects of dying, and the disabling effects of asthma in young people.

Michael Calnan is Professor of Sociology of Health Studies and Director of the Centre for Health Services Studies at the University of Kent. He has published extensively in the field of medical sociology and health policy and his recent books include a co-edited volume (with J. Gabe and M. Bury) *The sociology of the health service* (1991), *Preventing coronary heart disease: prospects, policies and politics* (1991), and (with S. Cant and J. Gabe) *Going private: why people pay for their health care* (1993). His current research interests include lay perspectives on health, illness and medicine, theories of medical power and the sociology of general practice.

Elaine Denny is Senior Lecturer in Nursing Studies at the University of Central England in Birmingham, where she is course director of a post-registration nursing degree. Her main areas of interest are health policy and women's health issues. Previous research has focused on family planning clinics and new reproductive technologies, and she is currently researching home nursing in mid-nineteenth century England for her doctoral dissertation.

Jonathan Gabe is a senior research fellow at Royal Holloway, University of London. He has published widely in the areas of mental health, health care professions, health policy and the mass media and health. He is co-editor of the journal *Sociology of Health and Illness*.

Uta Gerhardt is currently Professor of Sociology at the University of Heidelberg. Previous positions include the University of California, Berkeley, and the University of London (Social Science Research Unit, Bedford College). Her main fields of interest are sociological theory ("microsociology") and medical sociology. Her research has concentrated on qualitative approaches using ideal-type data analysis. Her main publications include a co-edited volume (with M. E. J. Wadsworth) *Stress and stigma* (1985), *Ideas about illness* (1989) and *Talcott Parsons on national socialism* (1993). Her empirical studies in the field of medical sociology have yielded two books in German: *Patientenkarrieren* (1986) and *Gessellschaft und Gesundheit* (1991).

Myfanwy Morgan is Reader in Sociology of Health at United Medical and Dental School, St Thomas' Hospital, and head of the social science section in the Department of Public Health Medicine. Her current research interests include patients' meanings and management of asthma, the significance of ethnicity for health promotion among Afro-Caribbean people, and illness behaviours and sickness absence among doctors and other professional groups. She has also published in the areas of disability and inequalities in health and on a range of health service issues, and is co-author of a textbook on medical sociology.

Alan Radley is Senior Lecturer in Social Psychology in the Department of Social Sciences, Loughborough University. His specific research interests are in the field of illness, though more generally in the body and social psychological theory. He is the author of several books, the most recent of which include: *Making sense of health and illness: the social psychology of health and disease* (1994), and an edited volume: *Worlds of illness: biographical and cultural perspectives on health and disease* (1993).

Lynda Rajan is a research associate at the Social Science Research Unit, Institute of Education, University of London. She has worked on a range of different projects, including (with Ann Oakley) the Social Support in Pregnancy study. Since then, most of her work and writing has been in the field of women's health and the maternity services, including an evaluative study of information giving and informed choice during pregnancy and labour.

Ursula Sharma completed her first degree in sociology and higher degrees in social anthropology from the University of London, and has drawn on both these traditions in her teaching and research. Her most recent research has been on complementary medicine in Britain and she is the author of *Complementary medicine today: practitioners and patients*. She is Professor of Sociology at the University of Derby.

Simon J. Williams is currently a Warwick Research Fellow and lecturer in the Department of Sociology, University of Warwick. Before that he was a Research Fellow at the Centre for Health Services Studies, University of Kent. He has published widely in the areas of the sociology of chronic illness, pain and disability, health and lifestyles, health promotion, and the lay evaluation of modern medicine and medical care. His current projects include a co-authored book (with G. Bendelow): *"Embodying sociology": critical perspectives on the dualist legacy*, and a co-edited international volume (with G. Bendelow) on: *Emotions in social life: social theories and contemporary issues*. He is also co-editor of *Medical Sociology News*.

Part I
Introduction

Chapter 1
Modern medicine and the lay populace: theoretical perspectives and methodological issues

Simon J. Williams & Michael Calnan

Introduction

How do lay people view modern medicine – a fountain of hope or a well of despair, an "illegitimate reification" or a "fixed point of reference" across a terrain of uncertainty? What criteria do they draw upon in evaluating differing forms of medical care and technology? And what does all this tell us about the relationship between modern medicine and the lay populace in the contemporary era? Are people, for example, simply passive and accepting, active and critical, or a mixture of both, and to what extent do views differ on the relative merits of modern medicine within the lay populace? Drawing upon a range of detailed qualitative and ethnographic research, these are some of the key questions that this volume seeks to address.

Essentially, the aims of this introductory chapter are threefold. First, we critically review some of the differing theoretical perspectives concerning the relationship between modern medicine and the lay populace. In doing so, we attempt to sketch the wider context within which lay perspectives and experiences of modern medicine take place. Secondly, having done so, we then proceed to discuss some of the methodological problems and empirical issues involved in research in this area. In particular it is argued that, in contrast to the growing number of consumer satisfaction surveys that litter the field, there is an urgent need for more detailed qualitative and ethnographic research within this area; research that seeks to unravel the complex, subtle and sophisticated processes involved in the lay experience and evaluation of modern medicine, and sheds further empirical light upon some of the more macro-focused theoretical debates. It is against this backdrop that the rationale for the present volume emerges. Hence, the third and final objective of this chapter is to discuss the nature and aims of the volume and briefly to introduce the chapters that follow.

2

Critical perspectives on modern medicine and the lay populace

Whether through the examination of lay concepts of health and illness (Blaxter 1983, Pill & Stott 1982, 1985, Cornwell 1984, Calnan 1987), the struggle between the voice of medicine and the voice of the lifeworld (Mishler 1989), or broader critiques of modern medicine as an institution of social control (Freidson 1970, Zola 1972), the relationship between modern medicine and the lay populace has been a source of considerable concern and debate for medical sociologists over the years. The conclusions reached, however, appear to differ considerably. For example, a number of theorists working at the macro-level (Parsons 1951, Illich 1976, Waitzkin 1979) have made the assumption that the public accepts the "efficacy" and legitimacy of modern medicine and therefore has complete faith in the value of scientific medical knowledge. Similarly, social historians tracing the development of modern medicine and the rise of the medical profession have suggested that during the nineteenth century, the public's views about scientific medicine were transformed from suspicion to a general acceptance (Larson 1978).

Certainly, it is true that from the middle of the nineteenth century onwards, healing changed from being a "rattlebag of quacks and rogues" (Porter & Porter 1989), to a profession with a considerable degree of power, status and authority (Gabe et al. 1994: xii). During this period, rapid advances in medical science confirmed the utility and legitimacy of the scientific perspective, and medical practitioners increasingly became "stabilising authorities within a world prone to occasional disorder" (Gabe et al. 1994: xii). In particular, Rudolph Virshow's "cell theory", together with the "germ theory" of Louis Pasteur, transformed medicine from an "art into a science" (Synnott 1993). These processes were subsequently carried forward in the first half of the twentieth century when significant developments occurred in the organization of medicine, the delivery of health care, and the scientific foundations of medical practice. Moreover, the Second World War also ushered in important political changes in Britain in the shape of the National Health Service and, following this, doctors' power and authority was further underlined by various other social, cultural and technological changes. In this respect, it has been suggested that doctors increasingly came to be cast in the role of "secular priests" whose authority and expertise encompassed not only bodily ailments but also prescriptions on a "good, virtuous and healthy life" (Gabe et al. 1994: xii). In addition, doctors also benefited from being the custodians of a whole range of new pharmacological products that were generally regarded by the public in terms of their life-saving qualities or their ability to minimize personal discomfort; a situation that was further enhanced in the 1950s and 1960s by surgical procedures such as organ transplantation (Gabe et al. 1994). As a consequence, the body became less an object of fear and more a source of enjoyment. This has led to an acceleration of the trend from sacred to profane attitudes towards the body in which: "the magic bullet now works better and quicker than prayer" (Synnott 1993: 28). Indeed, as Kelly and Field have recently argued:

> To deny the effectiveness of modern medical procedures such as coronary artery bypass, renal dialysis, hip replacement, cataract surgery, blood transfusion, the pharmacology of pain relief and the routine control of physical symptoms in restoring or improving the quality of life for those suffering from chronic illness is to deny the validity of the everyday experiences of the lay public in modern Britain. In stressing the limitations and costs of medical interventions, the physical and social contributions of modern medicine are all too frequently ignored (1994: 36).

In short, this line of argument suggests that, as a consequence of its historical struggle for professional status, together with significant and continuing advances in its knowledge base, methods of treatment and technological armoury, medicine has come to be largely accepted by the lay populace as a significant and legitimate authority within society, one that is formally backed and ratified by the state.

Others, in contrast, have suggested that the general public is becoming increasingly sceptical about the value of modern medicine (Strong 1979) and that, as a consequence, a radical rupture in societal trust is taking place. Much of the debate here has centred around the relevance or otherwise of the medicalization thesis. Hence, it is to a critical discussion of this debate that we now turn.

Medicalization, surveillance and control: the production of "docile bodies"?

Essentially, the concept of medicalization refers to the ways in which medical jurisdiction has expanded and now encompasses many problems that hitherto were not formerly defined as medical issues (Zola 1972, 1975). In the past two centuries a broad range of behaviours from homosexuality to alcoholism have been subsumed under the medical rubric, and the current obsession with locating the genetic precursors of diseases, disabilities and behaviours means that the knowledge base of scientific medicine has encroached still further into defining the limits of "normality" and the proper functioning, deportment and control of the human body (Lupton 1994). As Conrad & Schneider (1980) have pointed out, this process of medicalization can occur on a number of different levels: (i) *conceptually*, when a medical vocabulary is used to define a problem; (ii) *institutionally* when medical professionals confer legitimacy upon a programme or problem in which an institution specializes; and (iii) at the level of the *doctor–patient relationship*, when the actual diagnosis and treatment of a problem takes place. In addition, it has also been argued that a number of conditions need to be met before medicalization can occur. With regard to deviance, for example, it is suggested that this will only be medicalized if: (i) the traditional forms of social control are seen to be inefficient or unacceptable; (ii) the problem is associated, even if in a rather ambiguous form, with some underlying "organic" cause; (iii) the medical profession accepts the deviant behaviour as falling within its jurisdiction; and (iv) there exists some form of medical technology that can be used for social control purposes (Conrad 1981).

Yet, given this general consensus of opinion regarding the definition of medicalization, writers differ considerably concerning its causes. Some critics, for instance, have argued that the expansionist tendencies of medicine are primarily due to the medical profession exercising its power to define and control what constitutes health and illness in order to extend its professional dominance (Freidson 1970). Others, however, have considered medicalization to be the result of broader social processes to which doctors are merely responding. Thus according to Illich (1976), for example, the medical profession, as part of wider processes of industrialization and bureaucratization in society, has not only duped the public into believing that it has an effective and valuable body of knowledge and skills, but has also created a dependence through the medicalization of life that has now undermined and taken away the public's right to self-determination.

In contrast to the emphasis upon industrialization and bureaucratization in the process of medicalization, it has been argued that this phenomenon is a means of social control that serves the interests of particular powerful groups in society. For example, medicalization has been seen as serving the interests of the ruling capitalist class (Navarro 1975, 1986, Waitzkin 1979, 1983, Taussig 1980). Here, the creation and manipulation of consumer dependence upon medicine is seen as merely one instance of a more general dependence upon consumer goods created by that class. For others, however, medicalization is depicted as a form of social control that serves a heterogeneous array of interests such as institutions responsible for controlling deviance (e.g. prisons, schools and the family), the pharmaceutical industry, lay pressure groups representing deviants, as well as particular segments of the medical profession (Conrad 1981, Conrad & Schneider 1980, 1985, Gabe & Calnan 1989).

Feminists have also stressed the ways in which women's bodies and lives have become increasingly medicalized and subjected to control by a patriarchal medical profession. In particular, they have tended to pay most attention to those forms of medical technology that are experienced solely or mainly by women such as reproductive technology or psychotropic drugs. For example, it has been suggested that women experience childbirth as alienating not only as a consequence of the negative medical metaphors and images that pervade women's bodies (Doyal 1979, Scully & Bart 1978, Martin 1987), but also as a consequence of being coerced into accepting the use of obstetric techniques such as foetal monitoring, pain-killing drugs, induction and forceps without being told why such techniques are necessary or what risks are involved (Doyal 1979, Oakley 1980, Graham & Oakley 1981, Evans 1985, Tew 1990). In this sense, lacking control over what is a natural process, women may come to feel estranged from their bodies.

Certainly female reproduction in the late twentieth century is the subject of a number of contradictory and contesting discourses (Lupton 1994). Here, as Lupton (1994) suggests, the advent of IVF, embryonic transfer, surrogacy and ova and embryo donation, has provided a focal point for political struggles between feminism and medicine and has also proved to be the terrain upon which heated debate within feminism itself has occurred. Although some radical feminist writers have suggested that reproductive technologies are beneficial to women, others in contrast, have emphasized women's lack of choice in the face of male control over these new forms of reproductive technology (Steinberg 1990, Rowland 1992). In particular, it is argued that these new forms of reproductive technology reduce women's bodies to reproductive commodities and serve to further remove women's agency in the interests of patriarchal control. In this respect, medical scientists have been accused of experimenting on women for their own benefit rather than women's (Arditti et al. 1984). These perspectives have in turn begun to be challenged by post-structuralist feminists, who reject the notion that the "female body" is simply acted upon, instead viewing it as being an inscribed and socially constructed product of discursive processes (Sawicki 1991). As Lupton notes: "From this perspective the new reproductive technologies are themselves regarded as producing subjectivity rather than a 'false consciousness'" (1994: 158).

The emergence of poststructuralist feminist perspectives in turn resonates with Foucauldian perspectives on the social construction of medical knowledge and disease, which have also been influential in drawing attention to important elements of social control and surveillance that medicine exercises over our bodies and lives. For Foucault (1973), the medical view of the body that emerged towards the end of the eighteenth

6

century (i.e. the "clinical gaze") reflected broader changes and processes of rationalization that were occurring in society at that time (Turner 1984, 1987, 1992). Thus the view of the body as "something docile, that could be surveilled, used, transformed and improved", was evident not only in the context of the clinical examination within the hospital, but also in a wide range of other institutions including the prison, the asylum, the school and the military barracks. For Foucault, these institutions are depicted as important elements within an expanding apparatus of control (what he terms a "panoptic system of surveillance") that is predicated less upon the use of violence and more upon a micro-politics of disciplinary power; a "normalizing" power whereby individuals are morally regulated into conformity. In short, modern medicine is seen as part and parcel of a wider, more extensive, system of disciplinary techniques and technologies of power that are concerned with the moral regulation and "normalization" of the population through the medical gaze and regimen (Turner 1987).

Indeed, as Foucault argues in the *History of sexuality* (vol. I) (1979), life itself is now being occupied and regulated by medicine through both an "anatomo-politics of the human body" and the "bio-politics of the population". In other words, modern disciplines, systems of surveillance and control, and contemporary forms of knowledge/power are now increasingly focused upon the body and its reproduction (Turner 1987). Moreover, as Armstrong (1983) notes, the twentieth century has been marked not only by the consolidation of this "reductionist clinical gaze", but also by its extension beyond the confines of the clinic and the individual body and into its social spheres and spaces; processes that have been exacerbated by the recent advent of AIDS and the current emphasis upon health promotion, fitness and the "postmodern self" (Glassner 1989, Thorogood 1992, Armstrong 1993, Nettleton & Bunton 1993). Indeed, as Foucault himself acknowledged in his later writings, contemporary forms of control begin to move from panoptic-like structures to an emphasis upon what he termed "technologies of the self" (Foucault 1988).

In drawing upon this Foucauldian legacy, social constructionist perspectives on medical knowledge and disease have added yet another powerful challenge to the medical citadel and its preferred self-image as a scientific, morally neutral and value-free institution, predicated upon an altruistic concern for both patient and community welfare. Rather, according to these theoretical perspectives, a very different picture emerges; one in which medical knowledge is not simply timeless and a-historical, but grounded in specific socio-historical circumstances and forms of knowledge/power that determine its nature, content and form. In this sense medicine, as portrayed by social constructionists, is caught up in wider networks of disciplinary techniques and forms of surveillance that take the body of individuals and populations as both its subject and object. As

Bury (1986) notes, from such a perspective a question mark is certainly placed over the notion of "medical progress".

There are, however, a number of problems with these approaches. One of the common assumptions underpinning them is a portrayal of the individual or the lay public more generally as essentially passive and uncritical in the face of modern medicine's expansionist tendencies, whatever their source or origin. For example, as Turner (1987) notes in relation to the work of Foucault, given the power of discipline and surveillance, it is difficult to know how one could locate or explain opposition, criticism or resistance to medicine, or indeed any other form of dominance. Similarly, as Gerhardt (1989) has rightly observed, these approaches result in a largely "overdrawn" view of modern medicine and society that is seen to impose a "relentlessly forceful undemocratic order" (1989: 333) upon individuals. Certainly, as noted above, this is true of Foucault's early writings in which issues of discipline and control are dominant themes. Here the emphasis upon social control, the "fabrication" of scientific knowledge, and the supposed production of "docile bodies" appears, to say the very least, somewhat problematic, and there is a danger of exaggerating the hold that modern medicine has over contemporary experience. As Bury states: "allegations about the supposed negative effect of medical knowledge without adequate empirical checks as to its degree of negativity (or reification) is simply to perpetuate an argument without the possibility of refutation" (1986: 158–9).

From "docile" bodies to "reflexive" bodies: the "challenge" of the articulate consumer?

Partly as a consequence of these and other related problems, newer theoretical perspectives have begun to emerge that seem to cast a far more critical and accurate light on the changing relationship between modern medicine and the lay populace in the contemporary era.

Indeed, as a number of writers have suggested, the idea of general patient addiction or dependence on modern medicine is far too simplistic and not, in fact, based upon the everyday realities concerning the way in which the lay public thinks and acts in relation to health and illness (Strong 1979, Cornwell 1984, Crawford 1984, Kohler Riessman 1989).

For example, Cornwell (1984), in drawing on the work of Habermas (1971), makes a useful distinction between "traditional legitimations", which are tied to religious, philosophical and moral beliefs systems, and "modern legitimations" that are scientific and technical and founded upon empirical and analytical knowledge. Within this schema, the process of "rationalization" occurs as social life is transformed and traditional legitimations are replaced by modern ones. Moreover, this process of rationalization may occur at two different levels; first, at the level of culture as a whole (i.e. "rationalization from above"), and secondly at the individual and/or sub-cultural level (i.e. "rationalization from below").

As Cornwell argues, the advantage of using this conceptual framework for understanding the process of medicalization lies in the acknowledgement that

> the relationship of lay people to medicine, and thus by extension, to matters of health and illness more generally, can be analysed on different levels. It states the dominant tendency in our culture, which is towards modern scientific and technical forms of legitimation, without implying that the process will necessarily be carried through everywhere and in all social groups, at the same pace or at the same time. The rate of progress of medicalisation depends upon the state of readiness of the sub-culture and individuals within sub-cultures to allow it to take place, and on their state of awareness and knowledge of scientific achievements (Cornwell 1984: 120).

Similarly, Kohler Riessman (1989) has questioned some of the simplistic assumptions concerning the medicalization of women's bodies and lives. As she shows on the basis of historical and contemporary evidence, women have not simply been passive victims, rather they have been active participants in this process according to their class-based interests. As such they have both lost and gained as a result. Indeed, as Kohler Riessman argues, to cast them in any other light is to perpetuate the very myths and ideologies from which feminists have been trying to escape.

More generally, it is argued that increasing lay knowledge about modern medicine, declining deference to experts in society at large, changing attitudes of doctors, and changing patterns of morbidity are modifying social expectations concerning the doctor–patient relationship in the direction of mutual participation (Elston 1991). Moreover, some have even gone as far as to suggest that a radical rupture of societal trust, or a "de-medicalizing" of society (Fox 1977, Reeder 1978, Wikler & Wikler 1991, Lowenberg & Davis 1994) is taking place with a subsequent marked decline in medical dominance over patients and people's faith in professional mechanisms of self-discipline (Elston 1991). As Berliner suggests, discontent with modern medicine appears to be associated with the following factors:

(1) changes in the disease structure of modern societies; (2) changes in demographic patterns; (3) changes in the doctor–

physician relationship; (4) the limitations of the hospital; (5) problems associated with the technological approach to medicine; (6) the problems associated with the machine model orientation of scientific medicine; (7) the focus on cure over prevention in research and practice; and (8) the cost of medical care (1984: 40).

Indeed, as Lupton (1994) argues, western societies in the late twentieth century are characterized by people's increasing disillusionment with scientific medicine. Yet, paradoxically, there is also an increasing dependence upon biomedicine to provide the answers to social as well as medical problems, and the mythology of the "god-like physician" remains dominant: "On the one hand, doctors are criticised for abusing medical power by controlling or oppressing their patients, for malpractice and indulging in avarice; one the other, in most western societies, access to medical care is regarded as a social good and the inalienable right of every person" (Lupton 1994: 1). Moreover, as mentioned above, the fact that the populations of late twentieth-century western societies enjoy increased longevity and an existence more free of pain and physical discomfort than at any other time cannot be denied. In this sense, as Lupton suggests, medicine or faith in modern medicine is a sort of creed:

> There is a set of expectations surrounding health and the body prevailing in western societies: we expect to feel well, without pain or disability, long after middle age, we expect all children to survive birth and infancy, all women to give birth with no complications, all surgery and medical treatment to be successful. And for the majority of individuals these expectations are indeed met, serving to reinforce them even more strongly. However, although medical authority may confer an image of reassuring competence and control of the situation, the construction of the medical practitioner as omnipotent inevitably leads to disappointment and disillusionment when things go wrong, resulting sometimes in legal action against doctors . . . Furthermore, while we continue to look to medicine to provide help when we are ill, we also express resentment at the feelings of powerlessness we experience in the medical encounter (1994: 1–2).

Within all this, it is clear that the media play a crucial role in the "framing" and shaping of lay views and beliefs about modern medicine. More specifically, as Karpf (1988) suggests, the media may play *both* a "mystificatory" and "demystificatory" role. On the one hand, medicine and medical technology may be portrayed by the media through the use of "atrocity tales" concerning, for example, medical mistakes or tranquillizer dependence. Certainly, as Bury & Gabe (1994) have recently argued, the media may act as amplifiers and carriers of a critical and challenging position. On the other hand, the mass media may also be responsible for further mystification rather than demystification. Indeed, as Karpf (1988) argues, despite a greater number of critical programmes concerning medicine over the past decade, the media still largely portray medicine as the "triumphant conqueror of disease", in "miracle cure" reporting of heart transplants and test-tube babies.

In both Britain and the United States, patient and public voices have been most critical of medical science and practice in certain specific areas such as the management of reproduction (Oakley 1980, 1984, Evans 1985), chronic illness (Anderson & Bury 1988) and disability (Oliver 1990) where medicine has little to offer, and in areas of experimental treatment that arouse fundamental societal concerns such as transplant surgery or the new reproductive technologies (Elston 1991). Moreover, although Britain is not yet experiencing a medical malpractice "crisis" on the scale of that occurring in the United States (Annandale 1989, Dingwall 1994), it is nonetheless the case that recent years have witnessed a marked increase in the number of overtly expressed complaints concerning the quality of medical care through, for example, the NHS complaints machinery or civil actions for compensation (Elston 1991). Indeed, the recent introduction by the government of the *Patient's charter* (DoH 1991), coupled with the growing concern over the need to include "local voices" in purchasing decisions regarding health care (NHSME 1992, Popay & Williams 1994), is likely to further reinforce these trends. In short, as Gabe and colleagues have recently put it:

> In the last two decades the position of the medical profession appears to have changed. The corporate power of medicine has been increasingly challenged and doctors, the high priests of modern society, have become increasingly embattled as their position as experts has been challenged from inside and outside the health care arena. In conjunction with direct challenges to their knowledge and expertise have come doubts about the nature of their power, stirred by the secularisation of medical mystique and changing perceptions of the dynamics of power in society (Gabe et al. 1994: xiii).

Certainly, as Kelleher (1994) has recently argued, the growth of self-help groups can fruitfully be seen as a form of "lay resistance" to the dominance of medical instrumental rationality vis-à-vis experiential forms of knowledge. Similarly, the emergence of critical lay perspectives on public and environmental health issues poses a potentially significant epistemological and political challenge to conventional biomedical perspectives (Williams & Popay 1994), while the revival of anti-vivisectionist activity over the last 25 years provides a renewed challenge to medical science (Elston 1994).

In addition, recent years have also, of course, witnessed an important growth in the popularity of "alternative" or "complementary" therapies among the lay populace. As Sharma (1992) notes, resort to these various therapies is no longer confined to small groups of "enthusiasts". Rather, use of non-orthodox therapies is now widespread and popular in the broad sense of that word; something that, she suggests, poses a direct challenge to the authority of the orthodox medical profession, as well as raising important policy issues (Sharma 1992). Indeed, as Bakx (1991) suggests, western consumers are coming to distance themselves culturally from orthodox medicine perceived as arch-modernity personified; a phenomenon that in turn can be located within the broader socio-cultural and political framework of self-determination and a reclaiming of control over the body, self and wider environment (Coward 1989).

Yet as Lowenberg and Davis have recently argued, the "holistic health movement" contains within it elements that suggest processes of both demedicalization and medicalization. Thus whereas the locus of causality is restored to the individual and status differentials between providers and clients are minimized, suggesting processes of de-medicalization, the exponential expansion of the pathogenic sphere and the remit of the holistic health movement simultaneously suggest a drastic increase in medicalization. In this respect, echoing Armstrong's earlier critique (1986), Lowenberg & Davis (1994) suggest that the holistic health model subjects an increasing number of areas of everyday life to medical scrutiny and supervision due to its emphasis upon lifestyle modification and mind–body continuity. Seen in this light, the "liberatory" potential of alternative therapies and the holistic health movement takes on a more troubling hue. Moreover, at a broader level, as Saks (1994) suggests, although alternative therapies may pose important challenges to orthodox medicine, they have not, as yet, significantly reduced its dominance.

At a broader level, many of these issues are also raised in other recent theoretical perspectives stemming largely from America suggesting that the "challenge from the articulate consumer" is merely one strand in what is conceived of as a broader assault on medicine; a process that, it is claimed, is resulting in a gradual *"deprofessionalization"* (Haug 1973, 1988) or *"proletarianization"* (McKinlay & Arches 1985) of modern medicine. On the one hand, according to the deprofessionalization hypothesis, it is claimed that the popularization of medical knowledge through the media, increased literacy and the computerization of medical knowledge are combining to reduce the knowledge gap, undermine patients' trust in medical expertise, and increase their willingness to "shop around" for health care in the medical marketplace. On the other hand, according to the proletarianization theorists, members of the medical profession are being de-skilled, losing their economic independence, and being required to work in bureaucratically organized institutions under the instructions of a new cadre of managers, resulting in various forms of alienation similar to those experienced by the proletariat with the rise of the capitalist mode and relations of production. This, in turn, has sparked off a considerable debate as to the relative merits of these various new perspectives on professional power and dominance, together with their applicability in the British context (Freidson 1985, 1986, 1994, Navarro 1988, Elston 1991, Hafferty & McKinlay 1994, Gabe et al. 1994, Calnan & Williams 1995).

To summarize, contrary to earlier formulations, more recent theoretical perspectives stress that the lay public are not simply passive and dependent upon modern medicine, nor are they necessarily duped by medical ideology and technology. Rather, many forms of "counter-reaction" are beginning to emerge; responses that challenge any simple portrayal of the modern individual as passive in the face of modern medicine. Seen in this light, the notion of a "blanket dependence" on medicine or the fabrication of "docile bodies" appears to have a somewhat hollow ring to it, resulting in a largely "overdrawn" view of medical power, dominance and control.

Yet, beyond the level of theoretical speculation and broad social trends, what exactly do the lay public themselves think and feel about modern medicine and medical care, and what are the nature of their experiences in this domain? At present, with some notable exceptions, there remains a dearth of sociological research bearing upon these particular issues. Hence, it is to a further discussion of these empirical questions, together with a consideration of some of the methodological issues that they raise, that this chapter now turns.

The lay evaluation of modern medicine and medical care: from "consumer satisfaction" to "qualitative research"

In moving from the theoretical to the empirical level, it is clear that the lay evaluation of modern medicine and medical care has, until quite recently, largely been explored through studies of patient or consumer satisfaction. Generally speaking, such studies have tended to show that the vast majority of people and patients are happy with the services provided for them, although somewhat higher levels of dissatisfaction are found in relation to certain specific dimensions of care, particularly aspects of the doctor– patient relationship and the communication of information (Fitzpatrick 1984, Williams & Calnan 1992). As Fitzpatrick states, such evidence " . . . sharply challenge[s] any simplistic notion of a profound and widespread disenchantment with modern medical care" (1984: 162).

However, doubts about the reliability and validity of such findings have been a frequently voiced source of concern. This is so for a number of different reasons (Locker & Dunt 1978, Fitzpatrick & Hopkins 1983, Fitzpatrick 1984). The first problem concerns the fact that levels of criticism have been found to depend upon the way in which the questions are asked. It has been shown, for example, that less critical comments are given in reply to open-ended questions compared to more direct and specific questions. In addition, responses also appear to depend upon both the order and context in which the questions are asked (Judge & Solomon 1993).

A second problem concerns the uncertainty as to whether respondents' answers to questions correspond to their "real" views. Indeed, as Cornwell (1984) shows, there are strong social pressures and moral imperatives for people to express socially acceptable views when talking about health and health care. At a broader level, substantive empirical research has suggested that consumer satisfaction studies only portray a "surface" or superficial picture.

However, perhaps the most serious criticism of such studies relates to the general perspective and conceptual framework adopted and the topic areas included for investigation. As Fitzpatrick (1984) notes, despite widespread usage of patient satisfaction as a concept, there is little agreement as to its meaning. Indeed, Locker & Dunt conclude their review of the subject by saying that, "it is rare to find the concept of patient satisfaction defined and there has been little clarification of what the term means either to researchers who employ it or respondents who respond to it" (1978: 282). For example, Stimson & Webb (1975) found it difficult to categorize patients' responses to general practice consultations in terms of satisfaction. Rather, they suggest that patients' views fluctuate over time as they reappraise their consultation in the light of changes in their symptoms. More recently, Williams (1994) claims that patients may have a complex set of important and relevant beliefs that cannot be embodied in terms of expressions of satisfaction. In this respect he argues that for service providers to ascertain meaningfully the experience and perceptions of patients and the community then research must first be conducted in order to identify the terms in which those patients perceive and evaluate that service.

In short, the logic of these arguments suggests that it is, in fact, misleading to characterize such complex, changing views in term of "satisfaction" (Fitzpatrick 1984). Indeed, as writers such as Fitzpatrick & Hopkins (1983) have argued, the conceptual framework derived from patient satisfaction studies provides only partial and sometimes misleading insights into the perspectives of patients studied. For example, evidence from such studies has implied that patients very rarely evaluate medical care on grounds of clinical competence or expertise and very rarely evaluate modern medical practices such as the value of drugs or other aspects of technology. One possible explanation for this might be that patients, on the whole, do not have the knowledge to make such assessments and only acquire this knowledge in cases involving clinical conditions that require continuous and prolonged contact with doctors and other professional staff. Thus West (1976) for instance, in a study of doctor–parent encounters where the child was diagnosed as having epilepsy, showed that during the initial encounters parents were largely passive, uncritical and appeared satisfied. However, by the time of the third consultation, parents began to initiate questions themselves and forced information out of the doctor. The incompleteness of the information made available, along with the increasing knowledge and experience of the parents led them to become more critical and less satisfied and in some cases led to the threat of rejection of medical authority and expertise. This example clearly shows how satisfaction can change over time, particularly as a result of the acquisition of knowledge and experience by the patient or their representative. It also suggests that in certain areas of medicine, particularly where there is considerable clinical uncertainty such as with epilepsy or cancer (Calnan 1984), there is also perhaps the greatest potential for dissatisfaction among patients.

An alternative explanation for the scarcity of the type of evidence described above is that many studies of patient satisfaction have suffered from what may be termed a "managerialist bias"; that is to say, a domination by the providers' interests and perspectives rather than the patients' (Calnan 1988). Here, questions about the value of medical care and medical procedures as well as questions about the practitioners are rarely seen as appropriate for investigation in these studies. In other words these topics are rarely placed on the research agenda, at least in studies of patient satisfaction.

If a qualitative or ethnographic approach is used, however, a different picture emerges: one that highlights the complexity and richness of lay thought in this area (Fitzpatrick & Hopkins 1983, Calnan 1987, 1988, Calnan & Williams 1992, 1994, Gabe & Calnan 1989). In this respect, although large-scale surveys clearly have an important and continuing role to play in eliciting lay views and perspectives towards modern medicine and biotechnology (RSGB 1988, Macer 1994, Sanner 1994) – particularly if they manage to free themselves from the conceptual and methodological problems identified above – the nature of lay thought in this area calls for more detailed qualitative, or ethnographic research; studies that are likely to yield far richer insights and do justice to the complexity of the issues involved. This is an approach that attempts to understand the lay person's actions in terms of their own logic, knowledge and beliefs (Dingwall 1976). Hence, in contrast to studies rooted in the positivist tradition, the image of the lay person here is of one who is active and critical, who has his or her own complex system of theories about health, illness and medical care, who manages his or her own health requirements and who is discriminating in their use of medical knowledge, advice and expertise. As such, it is far more in keeping with the theoretical perspectives discussed in this chapter. Moreover, this commitment to qualitative, ethnographic research in turn relates to a more fundamental commitment to lay voices as the final arbiters in these broader theoretical debates centred around the (changing) relationship between modern medicine and the lay populace.

Yet with the notable exceptions of feminist research concerning women's experiences of medical care and technology (Oakley 1980, Evans 1985, Denny 1994) and sociological work on the experience of modern medicine in chronic illness (Anderson & Bury 1988), studies of a more detailed qualitative or ethnographic nature concerning lay perspectives and experiences of modern medicine and medical care are rare (Calnan 1987, 1988, Calnan & Williams 1992, 1994, Gabe & Calnan 1989). Moreover, as stated above, not only would such studies lead to far richer insights into these issues, they would also serve to ground many of the more abstract theoretical debates discussed at the beginning of this chapter.

It is in this context that the rationale and aims of the present volume emerge. In particular, as mentioned at the beginning of this chapter, the overarching aims and cohering themes of the book as a whole are as follows. First, to examine, on the basis of detailed qualitative and ethnographic work, the nature of lay perspectives and experiences of modern medicine across a variety of different contexts and social groups; secondly, to ascertain the criteria that structure the lay perception and evaluation of modern medicine; and finally, on the basis of this, to assess the extent to which modern medicine and medical care is coming to be questioned or challenged by an increasingly dissatisfied and critical lay populace. In this respect, the book aims to inform the more macro-focused theoretical debates surrounding modern medicine and the lay populace discussed earlier.

It should be stressed that "modern medicine", for the purposes of this particular book, refers to orthodox western medicine, and that medical technology, following Banta (1983), is taken to mean the drugs, devices, medical and surgical procedures used in medical care. In contrast, the definition of "lay" is rather more problematic. As Giddens (1994) suggests, "late" modernity is as an information-based society full of "clever" people. Moreover, as sources of knowledge pluralize and fragment, an expert in one area becomes a lay person in another. Nonetheless, for our purposes, "lay" can be defined as those members of society who, despite being potential "experts" in other areas, lack any formal or orthodox medical knowledge, training, qualifications or expertise. As such, the book aims to include both general public attitudes and opinions, and the experiences and evaluations of particular groups of patients in relation to specific forms of treatment, technology and care. In doing so, it spans a variety of differing levels of lay knowledge, experience and "expertise" concerning modern medicine, and seeks to examine the ways in which lay perceptions vary according to culture and social structure.

Essentially, the book is divided into five main parts. In the first part, we provide a general introduction to the volume as a whole. In particular, having sketched a theoretical backdrop to the volume as a whole in this chapter, Chapter 2 draws upon our recent empirical work in this area in order to examine the lay evaluation of modern medicine across a variety of different types of technology and contexts of care, including medicines and drugs, transplantation surgery and (new) reproductive technology. In addition, we also consider related issues such as faith in modern medicine and the nature of lay evaluative criteria regarding medical technology and "good" and "bad" doctors. Overall, these findings suggest a considerable degree of "ambivalence" among the lay populace; views that appear to differ according to which specific forms of technology are being considered (i.e. antibiotics, tranquillizers, hip replacements, heart transplants, etc.) and socio-demographic characteristics such as age, gender, class, educational status and health status. Thus, although doubt and scepticism are not uncommon, it is clear that the public continue to invest a considerable amount of faith in doctors and modern medicine. In this respect, lay thought appears to be structured around certain key dichotomies such as the following: "life saving–threatening", "quality of life enhancing–diminishing", "moral–immoral", "natural–unnatural", and "good–bad value for money". In addition, it is equally clear that, beyond their technical competence, the personal qualities and communication skills of the doctor are the attributes that are valued most highly among the lay populace. In short, these findings suggest a complex picture; one that casts considerable doubt on some of the more simplistic assumptions underpinning the medicalization thesis.

Medicines and drugs form a key component in modern medicine's technological armoury. Indeed, medicine may serve as a potent metonym for the doctor and biomedicine more generally. Consequently, the second part of the book examines lay views of a broad range of medicines and drugs. In Chapter 3 Nicky Britten discusses findings from a recent small-scale study concerning lay views of pharmaceuticals. In particular she distinguishes between what she terms "orthodox" and "unorthodox" accounts of medicines and drugs. Thus, although those giving orthodox accounts talked about medicine in a largely taken-for-granted, unquestioning fashion, those giving unorthodox accounts – the larger of the two groups – displayed far more of an "aversion" to medicines and did not seek medical legitimacy for their views. Here, common criticisms concerned the "unnatural" and "damaging" properties of medicines, and doctors were frequently criticized for "overprescribing". Given these views, "non-compliance" was a common response and, as Britten argues, it may constitute a key, albeit private, form of "resistance" to medical orthodoxy in "late" modernity.

In contrast, the next chapter by Jon Gabe and Michael Bury (Ch. 4) focuses specifically upon the social and cultural dimensions of "risk" in relation to tranquillizer use. In particular, drawing upon a range of data sources, they highlight lay people's risk perceptions of benzodiazepines, their management and attendant social risks, and the way in which these risks have been framed by the media's abiding interest in tranquillizers as a "newsworthy" issue. In keeping with previous chapters, they suggest that people have become more ambivalent about these drugs as the media have increasingly emphasized the risks of "addiction". However, despite widespread disquiet and media criticism, it is also clear that this ambivalence includes a measure of self-acceptance of tranquillizers and their role in everyday life. In this respect, they draw particular attention to the role of structural factors, such as gender, marital status, class, age and ethnicity and the way in which the absence of key social and material resources may override any negative perceptions of risk. It is this question of the relationship between structure and agency that, they suggest, needs to be more carefully examined in future work on the perception and management of risk in everyday life.

Finally, the last chapter in this part by Myfanwy Morgan (Ch. 5), examines lay views of anti-hypertensive medication with particular reference to ethnicity. In doing so, she draws attention to important cultural differences in levels of "adherence" to prescribed medication. However, rather than view the decision to "leave off" their medication as "irrational", Morgan is able to show how, through processes of "cultural reinterpretation" and the use of "traditional" folk remedies, the lower levels of "adherence" among the Afro-Caribbeans in her study can be readily understood as a "reflective" form of action that is grounded in their cultural beliefs and ways of life. Seen in these terms, not only does their familiarity with "natural" herbal remedies serve to emphasize the potency of modern drugs and thus contribute to their concerns, but the idea of "being on drugs" over a long period does not fit easily with their traditional notions of "cure" and "prevention".

Having considered medicines and drugs, the third section focuses upon the experience and evaluation of modern medicine and "life-saving" technology in chronic illness. Certainly this is an area where many of the potential problems and dilemmas involved in the meeting of medical and lay worlds come to the fore. In Chapter 6, Alan Radley examines the experiences of a group of coronary bypass patients and their spouses. In particular these experiences of surgery are considered in relation to certain critical junctures across the treatment trajectory, including the background to hearing of bypass surgery and the understanding of what it offered; expectations of treatment at the time of surgery and anticipation of the risks involved; the reactions to surgery some weeks after discharge, and finally, people's views on treatment one year later and their long-term reflections on what modern medicine had done for them. In doing so, Radley is able to show how couples embraced the prospects of improvement offered by this treatment and dealt with the possibilities of death in the course of the surgery. As he argues, in contexts such as these, it is simply not possible to evaluate medicine "at a distance". Rather, it "enters into" our everyday lives and personal biographies as much as it penetrates our bodies.

Continuing this theme of life-saving technology, the next chapter by Uta Gerhardt (Ch. 7), examines the experiences of medical treatment and patienthood in end-stage renal failure. Here, in a novel perspective, Gerhardt argues that the patient who receives the "gift of life" (i.e. live or cadaver-donor transplant), feels responsible for accomplishing as much "normality" as he or she can muster. In other words, if the individual is to "deserve" the gift received, then he or she is morally obliged to "prove" it by accomplishing as much of a return to normality as possible. In adopting this subtle perspective, Gerhardt is able to show how people's relationship to modern medicine is caught up in a complex web of moral imperatives and how patient careers and treatment options are hierarchically structured in terms of their legitimacy and desirability.

In contrast to life-saving technology, Chapter 8 by Gillian Bendelow moves us to the opposite end of the medical spectrum in charting the vicissitudes of hope and despair in chronic pain. Drawing upon a small-scale study of attenders at a pain relief clinic, she shows the complex interplay between people's styles of adjustment and their evaluations of medical treatment. For many of these patients, this was the "end of the road" and their last hope of finding relief. Unfortunately however, as Bendelow movingly shows, the all too common feeling was of medicine having "failed" them.

In addition to the chronically ill, women constitute another group whose lives, both historically and to the present day, have been intimately tied up with and controlled by medicine. Nowhere is this more so than in relation to childbirth and reproductive technology. Hence, the fourth part of the book includes two chapters, both of which critically examine women's own perceptions and experiences of reproductive technology. The first of these, by Lynda Rajan (Ch. 9), looks at women's experiences of pain relief during labour, their evaluations of its timing and effectiveness, and their feelings about "alternative" methods of pain relief. In addition, she also considers women's broader feelings about the nature and quality of the medical care provided in childbirth. In doing so, Rajan draws attention to the complex issue of "control" in this context, and demonstrates the subtle ways in which medical technology, far from reducing women's sense of control over the birthing process, may actually serve to enhance it. In this respect, women are not simply passive victims, but active participants in the medicalization process, and they stand both to gain and lose as a consequence.

These themes are further explored by Elaine Denny in Chapter 10 concerning women's views and experiences of in vitro fertilization (IVF). In particular, drawing upon a small-scale qualitative study of women undergoing treatment, she seeks to evaluate critically feminist debates surrounding the role of these new forms of reproductive technology. In this respect, she is able to show that although these approaches provide a partial explanation for the experience of some women, they neglect the extent to which these new forms of technology are actually seen by women themselves as a "resource" rather than a mechanism of social control or oppression. Indeed, as Denny argues, in treating women as universally oppressed and passive and failing to legitimate their own experiences, radical feminism, far from liberating women, provides an alternative source of oppression.

An implicit theme running through many of the chapters in this volume concerns the use of traditional remedies and complementary therapies. Indeed, much can be learnt about lay views of modern medicine through an examination of the reasons and decision-making processes involved in the use of complementary therapies and traditional remedies. Hence, this is a theme that is picked up and more fully addressed in the final part of the book. Here, Ursula Sharma, in Chapter 11, considers the growing popularity of "complementary" medicine among the lay populace and the potential "challenge" it poses to biomedical hegemony in late twentieth-century society. In particular, by drawing upon her own detailed research in this area, Sharma is able to show not only the attractions of "complementary" therapies, but also the continuing appeal of orthodox medicine. Indeed, as Sharma argues, rather than seeing these forms of therapy as a "countersystem", they may in fact display important elements of continuity with western biomedicine, and a key into contemporary cultural concerns with health and the preservation of the individual body in "late" modernity.

Finally, the volume closes with a brief conclusion, in which we seek to tie these diverse themes and issues together in the light of the three key questions posed at the beginning of the book. In particular, we seek to connect these issues up with broader social and cultural changes that are currently occurring in late modernity, such as the growth of social reflexivity, the emergence of active trust and radical doubt, and the re-skilling of the lay populace in the face of abstract systems of knowledge and expertise. In addition, on the basis of the evidence presented, we also sketch out a conceptual framework for the lay evaluation of modern medicine and medical care as a critical stimulus to further research in this area.

References

Anderson, R. & M. Bury (eds) 1988. *Living with chronic illness: the experience of patients and their families*. London: Hyman Unwin.

Annandale, E. 1989. The malpractice crisis and the doctor–patient relationship. *Sociology of Health and Illness* 11, 1–23.

Arditti, R., R. D. Klein, S. Minden (eds) 1984. *Test-tube women: what future for motherhood?* London: Pandora.

Armstrong, D. 1983. *Political anatomy of the body: medical knowledge in Britain in the twentieth century*. Cambridge: Cambridge University Press.

Armstrong D. 1986. The problem of the whole-person in holistic medicine. *Holistic Medicine* 1, 27–36.

Armstrong, D. 1993. Public health spaces and the fabrication of identity. *Sociology* 27(3), 393–410.

Bakx, K. 1991. The "eclipse" of folk medicine in western society. *Sociology of Health and Illness* 13, 20–38.

Banta, H. D. 1983. Social science research on medical technology: utility and limitations. *Social Science and Medicine* 17, 1363–9.

Berliner, H. S. 1984. Scientific medicine since Flexner. In *Alternative medicines, popular and policy perspectives*, J. Warren Salmon (ed.), 30–56. London: Tavistock.

Blaxter, M. 1983. The causes of disease: women talking. *Social Science and Medicine* 17(2), 59–69.

Bury, M. 1986. Social constructionism and the development of sociology. *Sociology of Health and Illness* 8(2), 137–69.

Bury, M. & J. Gabe 1994. Television and medicine: medical dominance or trial by media? In *Challenging medicine*, J. Gabe, D. Kelleher, G. Williams (eds), 65–83. London: Routledge.

Calnan, M. 1984. Clinical uncertainty. Is it a problem in the doctor–patient relationship? *Sociology of Health and Illness* 6(1), 74–85.

Calnan, M. 1987. *Health and illness: the lay perspective*. London: Tavistock.

Calnan, M. 1988. Toward a conceptual framework of lay evaluation of health care. *Social Science and Medicine* 27(9), 927–33.

Calnan, M. & S. Williams 1992. Images of scientific medicine. *Sociology of Health and Illness* 14(2), 233–54.

Calnan, M. & S. Williams 1994. The lay understanding of scientific medicine. In *The social consequences of life and death technology medicine*, I. Robinson (ed.). Manchester: Manchester University Press.

Calnan, M. & S. Williams 1995. Challenges to professional autonomy in the United Kingdom? The perceptions of general practitioners. *International Journal of Health Services* 25(2), 219–41.

Conrad, P. 1981. The discovery of hyperkinesis: notes on the medicalisation of deviant behaviour. In *Critical psychiatry: the politics of mental illness*, D. Ingleby (ed.), 102–19. Harmondsworth: Penguin.

Conrad, P. & J. Schneider 1980. Looking at levels of medicalization: a comment on Strong's critique of the thesis of medical imperialism. *Social Science and Medicine* 14A, 75–9.

Conrad, P. & J. W. Schneider 1985. *Deviance and medicalization: from badness to sickness*. London: Merrill.

Cornwell, J. 1984. *Hard-earned lives: accounts of health and illness from East London*. London: Tavistock.

Coward R. 1989. *The whole truth: the myth of alternative health*. London: Faber & Faber.

Crawford, R. 1984. A cultural account of "health": control, release and the social body. In *Issues in the political economy of health*, J. B. McKinlay (ed.), 60–103. London: Tavistock.

Denny, E. 1994. Liberation or oppression? Radical feminism and in vitro fertilisation. *Sociology of Health and Illness*, 16(1), 62–80.

Department of Health 1991. *The patient's charter*. London: HMSO.

Dingwall, R. 1976. *Aspects of illness*. London: Martin Robertson.

Dingwall, R. 1994. Litigation and the threat to medicine. In *Challenging medicine*, J. Gabe, D. Kelleher, G. Williams (eds), 46–64. London: Routledge.

Doyal, L. 1979. *The political economy of health*. London: Pluto.

Elston, M. A. 1991. The politics of professional power: medicine in a changing health service. In *The sociology of the health service*, J. Gabe, M. Calnan, M. Bury (eds), 58–88. London: Routledge.

Elston, M. A. 1994. The anti-vivisection movement and the science of medicine. In *Challenging medicine*, J. Gabe, D. Kelleher, G. Williams (eds), 160–80. London: Routledge.

Evans, F. 1985. Managers and labourers: women's attitudes to reproductive technology. In *Smothered by technology: technology in women's lives*, W. Faulkner & E. Arnold (eds), 109–27. London: Pluto.

Fitzpatrick, R. 1984. Satisfaction with health care. In *The experience of illness*, R. Fitzpatrick, J. Hinton, S. Newman, G. Scambler. London: Tavistock.

Fitzpatrick, R. & A. Hopkins 1983. Problems in the conceptual framework of patient satisfaction research: an empirical exploration. *Sociology of Health and Illness* 5(3), 297–311.

Foucault, M. 1973. *The birth of the clinic*. London: Tavistock.

Foucault, M. 1979. *The history of sexuality*, vol. I. Harmondsworth: Penguin.

Foucault, M. 1988. *Technologies of self: a seminar with Michel Foucault*, L. H. Martin, H. Gutman, P. H. Hutton (eds). London: Tavistock.

Fox, R. C. 1977. The medicalization and demedicalization of American society.

REFERENCES

In *Doing better and feeling worse*, J. H. Knowles (ed.). New York: Norton.

Freidson, E. 1970. *Profession of medicine*. New York: Dodds Mead.

Freidson, E. 1985. The reorganization of the medical profession. *Medical Care Review* **42**(1), 11–35.

Freidson, E. 1986. The medical profession in transition. In *Applications of social science to clinical medicine and health policy*, L. Aitken & D. Mechanic (eds), 63–79. New Brunswick: Rutgers University Press.

Freidson, E. 1994. How dominant are the professions? In *The changing character of the medical profession*, F. W. Hafferty & J. B. McKinlay (eds), 54–68. Oxford: Oxford University Press.

Gabe, J. & M. Calnan 1989. Limits to medicine – women's perceptions of medical technology. *Social Science and Medicine* **28**, 223–31.

Gabe, J., D. Kelleher, G. H. Williams (eds) 1994. *Challenging medicine*. London: Routledge.

Gerhardt, U. 1989. *Ideas about illness: an intellectual and political history of medical sociology*. London: Macmillan.

Giddeus, A. 1994. *Beyond left and right*. Cambridge: Polity.

Glassner, B. 1989. Fitness and the postmodern self. *Journal of Health and Social Behaviour* **30**, 180–91.

Graham, H. & A. Oakley 1981. Competing ideologies of reproduction: medical and maternal perspectives on pregnancy. In *Women, health and reproduction*, H. Roberts (ed.). London: Routledge & Kegan Paul.

Habermas, J. 1971. *Towards a rational society*. London: Heinemann.

Hafferty, F. W. & J. B. McKinlay (eds) 1994. *The changing character of the medical profession*. Oxford: Oxford University Press.

Haug, M. 1973. Deprofessionalization: an alternative hypothesis for the future. *Sociological Review Monograph* **20**, 195–211.

Haug, M. 1988. A re-examination of the hypothesis of physician deprofessionalization. *Milbank Memorial Fund Quarterly* **66**(Supplement 2), 48–56.

Illich, I. 1976. *Limits to medicine – medical nemesis: the expropriation of health*. Harmondsworth: Penguin.

Judge, K. & D. Solomon 1993. Public opinion and the NHS: patterns and perspectives in consumer satisfaction. *Journal of Social Policy* **22**(3), 299–327.

Karpf, A. 1988. *Doctoring the media: the reporting of health and medicine*. London: Routledge.

Kelleher, D. 1994. Self-help groups and their relationship to medicine. In *Challenging medicine*, J. Gabe, D. Kelleher, G. Williams (eds), 104–17. London: Routledge.

Kelly, M. & D. Field 1994. Comments on the rejection of the biomedical model in sociological discourse. *Medical Sociology News* **19**(2), 34–7.

Kohler Riessman, C. 1989. Women and medicalization: a new perspective. In *Perspectives in medical sociology*, P. Brown (ed.). Belmont, California: Wadsworth.

Larson, M. 1978. *The rise of professionalism: a sociological analysis*. Los Angeles, California: California University Press.

Locker, D. & D. Dunt 1978. Theoretical and methodological issues in sociological studies of consumer satisfaction with health care. *Social Science and Medicine* **12**(4), 283–92.

Lowenberg, J. S. & F. Davis 1994. Beyond medicalisation–demedicalisation: the case of holistic health. *Sociology of Health and Illness* **16**(5), 579–99.

Lupton, D. 1994. *Medicine as culture: illness, disease and the body in western societies*. London: Sage.

McKinlay, J. & J. Arches 1985. Towards the proletarianization of physicians. *International Journal of Health Services* **15**, 161–95.

Macer, D. R. J. 1994. Perceptions of risks and benefits of in vitro fertilization, genetic engineering and biotechnology. *Social Science and Medicine* **38**(1), 23–33.

Martin, E. 1987. *The woman in the body*. Milton Keynes: Open University Press.

Mishler, E. G. 1989. Critical perspectives on the biomedical model. In *Perspectives in medical sociology*, P. Brown (ed.). Belmont, California: Wadsworth.

Navarro, V. 1975. The industrialization of fetishism and the fetishism of industrialization: a critique of Ivan Illich. *Social Science and Medicine* **9**, 351–63.

Navarro, V. 1986. *Crisis, health and medicine: a social critique*. London: Tavistock.

Navarro, V. 1988. Professional dominance or proletarianization? Neither! *Milbank Memorial Fund Quarterly* **66**(2), 57–75.

Nettleton, S. & R. Bunton 1993. Sociological critiques of health promotion and the new public health. Paper prepared for: *Towards a Sociology of Health Promotion and the New Public Health Conference*: University of Teeside.

NHS Management Executive (NHSME) 1992. *Local voices*. London: NHSME.

Oakley, A. 1980. *Women confined: towards a sociology of childbirth*. Oxford: Martin Robertson.

Oakley, A. 1984 *The captured womb*. Oxford: Blackwell.

Oliver, M. 1990. *The politics of disablement*. London: Macmillan.

Parsons, T. 1951. *The social system*. London: Routledge & Kegan Paul.

Pill, R. & N. Stott 1982. Concepts of illness causation and responsibility: some preliminary data from a sample of working class mothers. *Social Science and Medicine* **16**, 43–52.

Pill, R. & N. Stott 1985. Choice or chance: further evidence on ideas of illness and responsibility for health. *Social Science and Medicine* **20**(10), 981–91.

Popay J. & G. Williams (eds) 1994. *Researching the people's health: social research and health care*. London: Routledge.

Porter, R. & D. Porter 1989. *Patient's progress: doctors and doctoring in eighteenth-century England*. Cambridge: Polity.

Reeder, L. G. 1978. The patient–client as consumer. In *Dominant issues in medical sociology*, H. D. Schwartz & C. S. Kart (eds). Reading, Mass.: Addison-Wesley.

Research Surveys in Great Britain (RSGB) 1988. *Public perceptions of biotechnology: interpretative report*. RSGB Ref. 4780 UK.

Rowland, R. 1992. *Living laboratories: women and reproductive technologies*. London: Pan Macmillan.

Saks, M. 1994. The alternatives to medicine. In *Challenging medicine*, J. Gabe, D. Kelleher, G. Williams (eds), 84–103. London: Routledge.

Sanner, M. 1994. Attitudes toward organ donation and transplantation. *Social Science and Medicine* **38**(8), 1141–52.

Sawicki, J. 1991. *Disciplining Foucault: feminism, power and the body*. London: Routledge.

24

REFERENCES

Scully, D. & P. Bart 1978. A funny thing happened on the way to the orifice: women in gynaecological textbooks. In *The cultural crisis of modern medicine*, J. Ehrenreich (ed.). London: Medical Review Publications.

Sharma, U. 1992. *Complementary medicine today*. London: Routledge.

Steinberg, D. L. 1990. Depersonalization of women through the administration of 'In Vitro Fertilization'. In *The new reproductive technologies*, M. McNeil, I. Varcoe, S. Yearly (eds), 74–122. New York: St Martin's Press.

Stimson, G. & B. Webb 1975. *Going to see the doctor: the consultation process in general practice*. London: Routledge & Kegan Paul.

Strong, P. 1979. Sociological imperialism and the medical profession: a critical examination of the thesis of medical imperialism. *Social Science and Medicine* 13A(2), 199–216.

Synnott, A. 1993. *The body social*. London: Routledge.

Taussig, M. 1980. Reification and the consciousness of the patient. *Social Science and Medicine* **14B**, 3–13.

Tew, M. 1990. *Safer childbirth? A critical history of maternity care*. London: Chapman Hall.

Thorogood, N. 1992. What is the relevance of sociology for health promotion? In *Health promotion: disciplines and diversity*, R. Bunton & G. Macdonald (eds). London: Routledge.

Turner B. S. 1984. *The body and society: explorations in social theory*. Oxford: Basil Blackwell.

Turner, B. S. 1987. *Medical power and social knowledge*. London: Sage.

Turner, B. S. 1992. *Regulating bodies: essays in medical sociology*. London: Routledge.

Waitzkin, H. 1979. A Marxian interpretation of the growth and development of coronary care technology. *American Journal of Public Health* 4(69), 1260–68.

Waitzkin, H. 1983. *The second sickness: the contradictions of capitalist health care*. New York: Free Press.

West, P. 1976. The physician and the management of childhood epilepsy. In *Studies in everyday medical life*, M. Wadsworth & D. Robinson (eds). London: Martin Robertson.

Wikler D. & N. J. Wikler 1991. Turkey-baster babies: the demedicalization of artificial insemination. *Milbank Quarterly* **69**, 5–39.

Williams, B. 1994. Patient satisfaction: a valid concept? *Social Science and Medicine* **38**(4), 509–16.

Williams, G. & J. Popay 1994. Lay knowledge and the privilege of experience. In *Challenging medicine* J. Gabe, D. Kelleher, G. H. Williams (eds), 118–39. London: Routledge.

Williams, S. J. & M. Calnan 1992. Convergence and divergence: assessing criteria of consumer satisfaction across general practice, dental and hospital care settings. *Social Science and Medicine* **33**, 707–16.

Zola, I. K. 1972. Medicine as an institution of social control. *Sociological Review* 20(4), 487–504.

Zola, I. K. 1975. In the name of health and illness: on some socio-political consequences of medical influence. *Social Science and Medicine* **9**, 83–7.

25

Chapter 2

Lay evaluation of scientific medicine and medical care

Michael Calnan & Simon J. Williams

As Chapter 1 suggests, the public's perception and assessments of modern medicine appear to be a neglected issue in sociological research. Moreover, views appear to differ on the relationship between modern medicine and the lay populace. At the theoretical level some macro-social theorists have portrayed the public as passively accepting that modern medicine is beneficial (Parsons 1951, Illich 1975, Waitzkin 1979). These theorists argue that patients either naturally accept the value of modern medicine or have been coerced or duped into accepting it (Calnan 1984). They have made the assumption that the public accepts that modern medicine is effective and thus has complete faith in the value of scientific medical knowledge. Similarly, social historians (Larson 1978) tracing the development of modern medicine and the rise of the medical profession, have suggested that during the course of the nineteenth century the public's views about scientific medicine were changed from suspicion to a general acceptance. Others, however, have been less concerned with the public's perceptions, as their theories suggest that power lies in the control over knowledge, and the practices and structures that sustain it. For example, Foucault (1973) suggests that the ways in which we perceive and speak about the body and medical matters is a product of wider historical conditions and power relations that shape and condition the knowledge base, and hence the prevailing mode of discourse in society at any given time.

More recently, macro-theorists have begun to suggest that transformations in "late" modernity have, among other things, increased the scepticism and critical perspective of the public as a whole, particularly in relation to the value of "experts" (Giddens 1991). Others, however, have suggested that the fit between the macro- and micro-levels is not as simple and neat as some of these theorists suggest and that this discourse of determinism leaves little room for issues of subjectivity and embodiment (Turner 1984). For example, Cornwell (1984) appears to have addressed this issue directly in her analysis of the process of medicalization. Cornwell draws on the work of Habermas (1971) who makes a distinction between what he terms "traditional legitimations", which are concerned with issues of human value that are tied to religious, philosophical and moral belief systems; and modern legitimations, which are scientific and technical and are founded upon empirical and analytical knowledge. The process of "rationalization" occurs as social life is transformed and traditional legitimations are replaced by modern legitimations (see Ch. 1).

The aim of this chapter is to present empirical evidence that throws light on the explanatory power of these different theoretical perspectives. However, before these data are presented it is necessary to consider how these issues have been examined empirically. At the empirical level, as Chapter 1 suggests, the most common approach to examining public views of health care has been mainly through general surveys of public opinion about health care and its financing and patient satisfaction studies, which with some exceptions show that patients are rarely critical of medical practice. This is in many respects surprising, given that some studies have highlighted the constant possibility of strain and tension in the doctor–patient relationship because of the many ways in which such encounters can prove unsatisfactory (Calnan 1984). One possible source of strain is that medicine cannot successfully solve all the problems with which it is presented. Yet, where criticisms are found, they usually focus on the personal qualities of the doctors or on their performance in the consultation, such as the ability to listen to patients' stories, to reassure, or to clearly communicate information about the patients' complaints (Calnan et al. 1994). Patients rarely, it appears, tend to be critical of the value of modern medicine.

This lack of patient criticism of medical practice and, to a greater extent, modern medicine may reflect either a high level of public satisfaction or lack of concern about medicine and medical matters. Alternatively, it might simply be an artefact of the perspective and methodology adopted (i.e. patients' views about medicine and medical practice may not have been an issue that was seen to be relevant or appropriate for the particular investigation, or was not given priority in the investigation). Also, the survey method may discourage the identification of critical comments through its use of structured questions that give little scope for articulation of "ambivalence" or critical thought (see Ch. 1).

In contrast, the studies and issues described here adopted qualitative methods to explore lay perceptions of medicine. The first study (Calnan 1988) involved tape-recorded interviews carried out in 1982 with women from working-class (10) and middle-class (10) backgrounds. All the women were married and had children and the sample incorporated a broad age range (21–55 years). The evidence presented here focuses on informants' discussion of the theme about faith in modern medicine as well as their evaluation of medical practitioners. This study raised a number of questions (not least whether the perceptions were gender specific) that were explored in a later study (Calnan & Williams 1992) carried out in 1988 and 1989. Once again qualitative tape-recorded interviews were carried out but this time with men and women who were married or living as married. The households were divided into ten couples from professional backgrounds and ten from manual backgrounds. The male partner was aged between 40 and 60.

The interviews in the later study had a more specific focus and explored informants' perceptions of a range of medical procedures including: antibiotics, heart transplants, test-tube babies, hip replacements, tranquillizers, vasectomy, hysterectomy and hernia. Also, once again questions were asked about their general faith in modern medicine. The aim of the selection was to attempt to span a broad spectrum of medical interventions that ranged from those of a more common everyday nature, such as antibiotics, to those of a high-technology life-saving nature, such as heart transplants, and those areas of more recent technological innovation such as test-tube babies. As the first study influenced the approach taken in the second study this chapter will discuss the themes and issues that emerged from both studies together. More specifically, analysis of the data from both studies will be used to identify the criteria used by lay people to evaluate modern medical technology.

Table 2.1 shows a typology illustrating the dimensions and criteria that emerged from informants' accounts to judge the value of modern scientific medicine and the range of technological procedures included in the investigation. The analysis will illustrate how these different criteria emerged by considering the different types of procedure in turn. It will also illustrate how a number of different criteria were used by informants to assess each of these procedures.

Table 2.1 Lay evaluative criteria.

"Good"	"Bad"
Life saving	Life threatening
Quality-of-life enhancing	Quality-of-life diminishing
Natural	Unnatural
Moral	Immoral
Necessary	Unnecessary
Restoring independence	Promoting addiction/dependence
Good value for money	Waste of money

Life-saving technology: the case of heart transplants

A range of criteria were used to evaluate heart transplants that reflected both the positive benefits as well as the negative aspects. In relation to the positive benefits it was the life-prolonging aspect that was emphasized. Those who emphasized the positive benefits tended to be men and working-class informants. First a middle-class man:

> Well, I think that if it can prolong someone's life, just for a few years possibly, and give them a better way of life for a short time, then they are a good thing.

And a working-class woman:

> Yes very good, it gives someone another lease of life, let's them live a bit longer, I'm all for that.

However, informants who were more ambivalent or critical evaluated heart transplants in terms of three other criteria. The first was a feeling that it was in some sense "unnatural". This is illustrated in the two following quotations:

> Well I don't think you have a normal life afterwards . . . You have got to take drugs and the fear of rejection, that is kept very, very quiet I think, and I think it is still in the experimental stage at the moment.

The second theme was associated with the religious, ethical and moral dilemmas involved. For example, a working-class woman stated:

> I can't honestly say, probably if I needed one I'd be all for them. It's a very peculiar feeling I get, but I don't like the idea of them . . . I don't mind kidney transplants but the heart . . . Perhaps, it's sort of semi-religious. I really don't know, its a bit sacrilegious.

Whereas a working-class man remarked:

> I'm a bit unsure of this. I had one of those donor cards that you carry around and I sat and looked at it and read it, and then I didn't sign it. It's a good thing, but there was a case on the radio today. Britain's youngest heart transplant, well it's alright providing its going to be alright for her. But if it's kept her going for something else to go wrong and mess her up for the rest of her life would they have been better leaving her as she was?

The issue of age could also be included under this criteria. For example, a working-class woman stated:

> Not wishing to sound cruel, but I think heart transplants on younger people are more valuable than on older people . . . I feel that a man of 65 or over who has had a good life, we accept that their time comes, but we don't accept that with a child of nine.

Finally, the third theme to emerge from the accounts was that of economic cost and the management of finite resources within a health care field of competing needs and priorities. For example, one middle-class woman stated:

> If I had a husband who needed one, I'm sure I would be very positive, and I know that this is a very selfish attitude for me to take, but overall I think too much money is spent in this area and not enough in routine care.

This issue of resource allocation relates to the previous one concerning the moral and ethical dilemmas of organ transplantation surgery. Moreover, as these quotes suggest there was an important difference in attitude between, on the one hand, people's general attitudes and orientation towards this procedure, and their views if the circumstances involved a loved one.

Medicine and drugs: an anti-drug culture?

The informants in the earlier study (Calnan 1988), particularly the working-class women, tended to focus their greatest criticism of medical technology on medicines and drugs and there was some evidence of an anti-drug culture as the following informant suggested:

> Well the stuff we swallow? Well a lot of it I don't agree with and I would rather go without but there again, if the children are ill, I would rather go to the doctor and get something for theirs, but for myself I would rather suffer or take something that I know like dispirins or whatever.

Certainly, this study showed that the greatest criticisms focused on the use of drugs, whereas procedures such as heart transplants and kidney machines were believed by the majority to be making an important contribution. Hence, in the second study the issue of an anti-drug culture was explored more fully by focusing on informants' evaluation of two different types of prescribed drugs: antibiotics and tranquillizers.

Antibiotics

Informants from the first study expressed concern about the over-prescribing of antibiotics.

> Some of it, OK, its fair enough, but I think a lot of it has gone on a bit too far. A bit too advanced. Penicillin I think is not given out correctly and is given out by some people as if it's aspirin. Some doctors give it out like aspirin and yet we found with the grand-daughter, she suffers from a bad cold or cough, and she needs something extra and she's given cough linctus. You know, so, sometimes I wonder if its worth getting any medication at all or just going along and letting things take their course.

The informants in the second study generally expressed positive opinions with respect to antibiotics but, as in the previous study, there was a frequently expressed caveat, namely that antibiotics were all right provided they were not "abused" or "overprescribed", as due to the risk of immunity, their efficacy would decline. This issue appeared to be more often raised by women rather than men and middle-class informants rather than working-class informants. For example, this was a response from a middle-class woman:

> Well, I mean antibiotics have revolutionized treatment haven't they?
>
> Interviewer: In what way?
>
> Well because people just died by the score didn't they, but antibiotics now enable people to live longer.

The question of "over-usage" or "abuse" was again well illustrated by a middle-class woman.

> If they are not abused and used in moderation, yes . . . we've got a great problem if they are abused because that means we have got to go on and develop new types of antibiotics, because the more frequent penicillins have been abused and bacteria have become immune to them.

In general, therefore, antibiotics were seen to be beneficial when used in "moderation" and they were judged in terms of their good and bad effects on illness and its control.

Tranquillizers

In contrast to antibiotics there was evidence of strong anti-tranquillizer culture among the lay population. None of the informants were wholly positive in their evaluation of tranquillizers. The negative or ambivalent feelings expressed about tranquillizers illustrated that tranquillizers were evaluated in terms of their propensity to induce "addiction" or "dependency", that they were unnecessary and were prescribed too frequently. First, the concern that they were or could be addictive was well illustrated by the following working-class informant:

> No, I don't believe in tranquillizers, not really. Well they can get a hold on you and trying to get off them is very, very hard, if you can do without I would say, yes, do without.

The second reason was that they were given too frequently as a working-class woman stated:

> They are addictive. I don't care what you say, and if it keeps the patient quiet, then I think the doctors issue them willy-nilly. I mean, when I was having problems with Andrew, Doctor W said to me, You know, I can put you on tranquillizers. But I said, oh no, I could not have that, well they don't make the problems go away, they just dull them don't they?

This last quotation also illustrates the third explanation, in that tranquillizers made the problems more tolerable, but did not usually deal with the root cause.

These strongly negative attitudes tended to be expressed more frequently by the working-class informants although the ambivalent attitudes by the middle class also included these negative aspects of tranquillizer use. However, they also tended to stress that they did have a place or function in certain specific cases – such as short-term management cases – if used prudently and monitored closely. For example a middle-class woman said about tranquillizers:

Only in extreme cases. I doubt they solve the problem that is causing the need for them. You have got to get to the bottom of the
problem. I don't think they are a good idea, only in extreme cases.
Maybe you have a bereavement and something drastic has happened to you and you need a little help for a little while, well
maybe it's OK but not the way they are doled out year-after-year.

Elective surgery

Hip replacements and hernia operations were the elective surgical procedures explored and similar criteria were used to evaluate both.

Hip replacements

This particular form of medical technology was one of the most highly
regarded and praised for its intervention, possibly because its benefits
were readily apparent in terms of reducing pain and suffering, increasing
mobility and improving the quality of life of these recipients. This perception was evident in most informants' accounts irrespective of class or
gender. For example, this is well illustrated in the comments of a working-
class man:

> Yes great . . . well my mother in law, she's had two done and see-
> ing the pain and agony she was in before, I think they are doing
> absolute wonders for the patients who need them. Yes, I think its
> wonderful.

Similarly a middle-class man remarked:

> I think they are a very important operation. A lot of patients have
> had a revived lease of life from the operation.

Indeed, the only note of dissent, came from a middle-class man:

> I have not known personally anybody who has had a completely
> successful hip operation, they really don't seem to be that comfort-
> able afterwards.

Hernia operations

As with hip operations, it seemed that the benefits of hernia operations were readily apparent; mitigating pain and suffering and improving the person's quality of life. For example, a working-class man dramatically remarked:

> Well I look on that the same way as I do hip operations, without them I think we would be lost. Yes, I think the medical people and people who pioneered such operations, they have done a lot of good to mankind.

Whereas a middle-class woman remarked:

> Oh yes, I think hernia operations for those who have the problem are very good and I wouldn't have thought they were tremendously expensive operations. I think it is a great shame that very many people have to wait months on some occasions to have one done.

Reproductive technology

Hysterectomy, vasectomy and test-tube babies were the reproductive technological procedures explored and each procedure was generally perceived in a different way although similar lay criteria for assessment were in evidence.

Hysterectomy

The benefits of hysterectomy were well accepted, particularly in terms of improvement in the quality of life; for example, a working-class woman said:

> That's the womb being taken out isn't it? If its diseased. Yes. I believe in having it taken away.

And a middle-class woman stated:

> I would say, yes, because I've got so many friends who have had them and are living such a much better quality of life, so I would say yes.

There were, however, a small number of middle-class women who expressed certain qualifications, particularly in terms of whether it was really necessary:

> If it's really, really necessary. A lot of it is only done you know, people have hysterectomies who really can't be bothered with the change, you know, you hear these stories, and in certain cases, such as with cancer you've got no choice.

Vasectomy

The question of whether a particular medical procedure was really necessary also emerged in the context of informants' discussion about vasectomy. This was expressed by a group who represented about half of the informants who might therefore be described as "ambivalent" about this procedure. For example, a middle-class man stated:

> They are sort of unnecessary really, unless its essential. I don't know of any essential indications for a vasectomy.

While a working-class man remarked:

> Well I suppose they serve a purpose. I mean I'm not against birth control and things like that as such, but I mean there are other forms of birth control without vasectomy, I think its a bit over-drastic.

In contrast, the other group of informants all emphasized the positive aspects of this procedure with comments such as the following:

> Well I think its probably a good thing I suppose.

> Well I suppose it solves any unwanted babies or that sort of thing.

Test-tube babies

A number of interesting themes emerged in informants' evaluation of "test-tube" babies. One of these concerned the benefits for couples who could not have children. For example, a working-class woman stated:

> Well, I think there are a lot of couples in the world who would like to have children but can't, so, yes its a help isn't it.

And a middle-class woman shared a similar view:

> Yes, yes I think if a couple really long for a child, and this is the only way they can do it, yes.

Other themes emerged among a second group of people who were more ambivalent about this form of technology. For example, there was the suggestion that it was in some sense "unnatural" and that it was a bad thing that could be "taken too far". For instance, a working-class man stated:

> I don't altogether believe in that, I don't like it at all. I think it should be a natural function between two parties, not done artificially in a test tube.

Whereas a middle-class woman remarked:

> There again, its all right for me, I've got five. If I had got no children then maybe I would go to any lengths to get a child and that would be quite acceptable. I think in moderation, but again it can be taken too far, genetics is a dodgy business.

As before it was clear that there was a division between general attitudes concerning the issue of test-tube babies and people's opinions if their circumstances were different and they were childless. Again the issue of the cost of such technology was also stressed, compared with other competing needs and priorities.

Evaluation of medical practitioners

In the first study (Calnan 1988) lay perceptions of medicine not only focused on medical procedures but also included evaluation of medical practitioners (i.e. family doctors). Each respondent was asked to assess their own family doctor in terms of whether they considered them to be "good" or "bad" and to explain why they made that particular assessment. Depending on the answers, further questions were asked, when necessary, about what the respondent understood to be a good and a bad family doctor. It was possible to identify from these series of questions the criteria that respondents used to assess their family doctors.

The criteria used by women from both groups to assess what is a good and a bad family doctor are shown in Table 2.2. While both groups of respondents identified a wide range of criteria, only the most frequent are presented in the table. Many of the criteria frequently used by both groups

Table 2.2 Patients' criteria for evaluating their family doctor. Criteria, in order of importance.

	Social Classes I, II	Social Classes IV, V
"Good doctor"	Sympathetic	Gives a lot of time
	Knows them personally	Treats children well
	Immediately refers to specialist	Listens
	Examines thoroughly	Examines thoroughly
	Gives a lot of time	Friendly
"Bad doctor"	Routinely gives prescriptions	Does not listen
	Treats everything as a waste of time	Routinely gives prescriptions
	Will not make house calls at night	Abrupt/rude manner
	Does not listen	Uncaring

were similar: gives a lot of time, examines thoroughly, and listens to the patient's story were common. The following examples illustrate these criteria:

> I personally like my doctor because he doesn't rush you and write out a prescription . . . . you have to wait but when you do see him he will listen to you.

> One that sits down and listens until you have finished speaking, instead of interrupting, writing out a prescription before you have finished. If you have got a sore throat, he should look at your throat and things like that and if you have got any pains in the chest or anything like that I think they should send you to have an X-ray, but he says, "I will give you painkillers" and that's about your lot. Of course, he doesn't think it is anything too serious. But I think a good doctor is one that sits down, listens to what you have to say, and has got a smile on his face now and again, you know, not like the one I've got, and one that gets on well with children.

> A caring doctor that will take the time to find out what is wrong. One who is as quick to listen as he is to examine.

> He's very caring and thorough and extremely kind. He gives me time when I go and never rushes me . . . he spends a long time trying to get to the root of the problem.

The women from the different social class groups, however, did identify some different criteria in their assessments. Women from Social Classes IV and V were particularly concerned about the manner of the doctor: good doctors were friendly and bad doctors had a rude and abrupt manner. The doctor's manner with children was also important, as the following respondent illustrated:

> Sometimes, let's say, sometimes he is and sometimes he isn't Em . . . he's a very abrupt man, he frightens the life out of you to start with so you don't go there unless . . .
>
> Interviewer: How does he frighten you?
>
> Er . . . he's very abrupt and he'll shout and holler at you and he'll swear at you occasionally but he's good with children.
>
> Interviewer: In what way?
>
> He's good with them . . . often children will go there and they're frightened of the doctor which is natural and he will reassure them. And he's good tempered with them, he doesn't always in my mind treat them best but he's a fair doctor – let's leave it at that.
>
> Interviewer: Why do you think your previous doctor was lovely?
>
> Well he was because when my daughter was a baby and she was very chesty, and stuff was hard to get then, and I used to go to him and nothing was too much trouble for him, and he'd put her on good things to clear her up, and he used to give me anything. And he took time with the kiddies, and although I did not go to him a lot you used to go into his surgery and he'd know you straight-away – your name. And he was an Indian, you know, and I used to well, you know, I was a bit prejudiced really I suppose but he was a really good doctor.

In contrast, women from Social Classes I and II put greater emphasis on two other aspects. First, the speed with which the doctor is willing to refer them or their families to hospital specialists:

> Now my last doctor, he was a nice man, but I wouldn't say he filled me with great confidence in everything. But he was very good in that he would always send you to hospital to see some-body if he didn't know, which I think is a good thing. I mean I'm always pleased when they send me to a specialist.

Secondly, the importance of having a sympathetic and reassuring doctor was also referred to by this group as a particular criticism of some doctors who made them feel that they were wasting their time. This is well illus-trated by the following respondent:

He doesn't make you feel that you're there unnecessarily, and whereas lots of doctors will prescribe drugs on letter and demand, our present doctor will only give my father-in-law a month's supply and then he wants to see him to take checks, blood pressure and examine his chest and back. And I think this is very good because it is not every doctor that will take that sort of trouble.

The difficulty in persuading doctors that the patient's complaint is serious is well illustrated by the following respondent, also from Social Classes I and II:

Yes, I think he is a good doctor but he is far too busy to have much time to spend with anybody, but he is basically a very good doctor. Yes, especially if you really have got something wrong with you, but unfortunately I think he spends most of his time dealing with people who haven't and it is very difficult sometimes to persuade him that you actually have got something wrong with you. But I think that having said that, I think he is a good doctor.

The criteria used to assess bad doctors were similar to those used to assess doctors as good. Not listening was a common complaint among both groups. Having an abrupt manner or being rude was specifically referred to by the working-class women, and treating patients as if they were "wasting the doctor's time" was one specifically referred to by the middle-class women. The routine use of prescriptions was also commonly referred to by both groups, as the following examples illustrate:

A doctor who didn't care very much, hasn't got any time for you and just writes out prescriptions and that.

Well, them that don't care about you . . . they just sit you down and write out a prescription for you before you've said anything – so they tell me.

Oh yeah and he was very rough. You used to walk into his surgery and your name and address would be on his pad before you've sat down. I'm telling you, he did not even question you . . . I didn't get on with him at all.

Somebody who will prescribe drugs of any sort, even antibiotics, without just cause. In some cases without even seeing the patient . . . takes too much responsibility on himself without referring to another person . . . who wouldn't come out at night if there was an emergency.

I haven't a lot of confidence because she's not very impressive . . . she seems to be a routine questioner and a routine prescriber.

In summary, while some emphasis was placed on the clinical competence of the doctor – carrying out a thorough examination or referral behaviour – women on the whole tended to emphasize the personal qualities of the doctors or their style in the actual consultation. Again, the routine use of prescriptions was a major source of criticism, not just because people were sceptical about the value of drugs, but because it produced a poor social relationship between themselves and their doctor.

Faith in modern medicine

This general question was explored in both studies and although there was a considerable degree of faith in modern medicine and technology as a whole, the working-class women in the first study expressed more scepticism, particularly about drugs, than the middle-class women. The second study, however, revealed no evident class difference, although women tended to be more ambivalent or critical than men.

The discussion of faith in medicine identified similar themes to those discussed earlier but also some new ones. For example, there was evidence of the positive side of medicine, but as this working-class informant suggested there was also concern about drugs:

Well I'm a very anti-drug person, I don't like taking drugs for the sake of it, which I tend to feel is what my doctor does sometimes . . . So therefore I don't think medicines help a great deal. As far as other respects well I haven't really had any dealings with . . . apart from a couple of years ago when I had this problem with my eldest daughter you know. And it was marvellous to be able to, you know, when she came home from the cardiac unit and she told me all what they'd done and how they done it. I mean, that they just could not have done that a few years ago. So in that respect I think, you know, with the transplants and everything that they're doing . . . never heard of it in my younger days. So . . . I think that the medical research that is being done is probably . . . a good thing yeah.

Thus, although this informant expressed ambivalence about modern medicine's achievements in terms of the side-effects or limited effectiveness of drugs she nonetheless appreciated the value of high-technology medicine in the treatment of heart disease. Similarly, the following informant not only expressed the benefits of high-technology medicine but also its limits:

> Oh well yes, now kidney machines I think they are really good. I mean they do their job, they recycle blood and that must be good, so that sort of technology, yes. Micro-chips, in years to come, well we will be able to do a lot more with them. You know, they've just put out this typewriter with micro-chips in it to help the deaf, like a typewriter, and they can hear. Now that is good. Things like that, but as for them researching on this cancer thing, well, I say they have wasted a lot of money. I don't know whether people would agree that they have wasted it. They have not found a cure yet and I mean that it could go on for years and years and years, doing this research . . . they should put more money into the things they know do work, I mean, like kidney machines.

Certainly this informant identified the need for value for money, although the failure of modern medicine was clearly illustrated through the example of cancer that was a recurring theme in other informants' accounts:

> In short . . . not a lot of faith. Some things they've done a lot for . . . like the things they can cure, but as for the rest like cancer and so on . . . well I think there's too much experimentation going on to my liking . . .

Finally, two other themes emerged in relation to medical interventions. One was the impossible task that medicine had set itself:

> I think we can go on perfecting various ways of combating illness but I don't think we will ever get there myself . . .

and the other was the social or human aspects of medical technology. This latter issue was well illustrated in the following informant's account of her experience of intensive care units:

> The way they treat patients for health reasons is good but the way they actually treat the person, what I mean . . . psychologically it does more damage than the actual disease, that's my view anyway. They do a lot for their patients, they'll fight and fight and fight until the bitter end but it's gone a bit too far and they've left one person behind . . . I mean the person as a person has been forgotten. You're just a number, or a carcass if you like.

Discussion: implications for theory and research

In turning to a discussion of the findings from the two studies a number of issues and points emerge. The first study initially set out to find if some of the macro-theorists were accurate in the way they portrayed the public and patients in their theoretical accounts of the position of modern scientific medicine. The simplistic assumption that the public and patients uncritically accept (for whatever reason) the value and benefits of modern medicine is, according to the evidence from the first and the second study, inaccurate. Instead, as the findings show, perceptions differ on the relative merits of modern medical technology according to which specific forms of technological intervention are being considered. The results also show that these medical technologies are evaluated according to the range of differing criteria that were outlined in Table 2.1.

Theoretically then, if the medicalization thesis is too simplistic and thus has limited explanatory power what other theoretical perspectives provide a more powerful explanation? The ambivalence about modern scientific medicine found in these studies may be explained by Cornwell's (1984) approach discussed earlier (see also Chs 1 and 3) that distinguishes between the macro-level of rationalization from above and rationalization from below. It is clear that rationalization from below has indeed occurred, at least at the level of lay beliefs. However, it is also clear that concerning certain aspects of modern technological medicine, this rationalization seems incomplete. Thus, for example, although hip replacements were whole-heartedly endorsed by the lay populace, tranquillizers, heart transplantation surgery and test-tube babies seem to be in opposition to certain cherished moral beliefs and values.

The question is whether these beliefs are a product of traditional values or are a product of other, more recent changes either in medical ideology or in other social and economic conditions at the macro-level that have influenced the structure of lay thinking and encouraged a degree of ambivalence or scepticism about scientific medicine among the lay populace. Certainly, there is evidence to suggest that these beliefs are at least in part a product of traditional values, in that work carried out on elderly populations (Calnan 1989) shows that, as with their younger counterparts, there was a strong anti-drug culture. These studies of elderly people have shown that while patients accepted doctors' prescriptions for medicines, the patients never actually used them and they were normally discarded.

This, however, may only provide a partial explanation in that rationalization and medicalization from above may also be undergoing a change. For example, 20 years ago the value of modern scientific medicine might have been less in doubt than it is now. Scientists are no longer the gods that they once were and there is some evidence of disunity in the scientific community, although perhaps less so among the more tightly knit medical profession. However, at least in the United States, it has been argued that professional medical autonomy is under threat from a more knowledgeable and enlightened consumer (Haug 1988). This enlightenment and the demystification of science and scientific medicine may partly have been brought about by the mass media who may on the one hand dramatize the success stories such as heart transplants and test-tube babies, and on the other amplify the atrocities and limitations of scientific medicine and its practice. Thus, the ambivalence expressed by respondents in these studies may reflect, at least in part, the impact of this demystification process.

The question of how far beliefs are products of traditional or contemporary values also is apparent in relation to the natural/unnatural theme that emerged in the context of discussion about test-tube babies. In this way an estrangement from nature and the natural course of life processes and production is seen to be a bad thing: bad that is from the traditional viewpoint of, to coin a phrase, "letting mother nature take its course". On the other hand the increasing numbers of the lay population who are turning to complementary forms of medicine and healing may symbolize an estrangement from and increasing awareness of the limitations of scientific medicine and dissatisfaction with its narrow biomedical focus.

A similar set of points can be made in relation to the issue of morality. In an increasingly secular world where science and rationality have to a large extent replaced religious and metaphysical systems of belief, there appears, at first sight, to be little room left for those more traditional legitimations (Habermas 1971). Yet again, as our data suggest, the dispassionate rationality with which science and scientific advance are associated leads it into issues that clash head on with fundamental religious, moral and ethical beliefs. Hence, the ambivalent or critical attitudes sometimes expressed towards certain forms of technological innovation such as heart transplants that in a sense were seen to be immoral. In this respect the removal of the heart was seen as "sacrilegious" as it was a sacred object and the very core or essence of a person.

At another level, the data also illustrate the differing sets of beliefs held by individuals according to whether the particular procedure under consideration relates to them or their family personally, or to members of the public in general. To some extent, this may reflect the analytical distinction which Cornwell (1984) draws between public and private accounts. In particular, public accounts in this context may be characterized by a general ambivalence about various forms of modern technology whereas private accounts may be less concerned with wider issues of public principle and morality, and instead have a more self-interested focus. However, in this respect the content of public accounts may actually differ

43

somewhat from that suggested by Cornwell, in that they may not simply reflect or reproduce dominant medical ideology but, instead, may stress traditional beliefs and ambivalence. This parallels the issue about the different perceptions of those who have gained knowledge through direct experience of the technology and those whose knowledge is derived from more indirect sources such as the media. Those who experience the procedure may use this to shape their views whereas those who have no direct experience may be influenced by the broader ideological messages that are filtered through the media (Karpf 1988; see also Ch. 4).

There was also some evidence, at least from the first study, of a connection between informants' judgements about scientific medicine and their criteria for assessing medical practitioners. This connection was found in relation to the routine prescribing of drugs, a practice that was considered to be doubtful from a therapeutic point of view and suggested also that the doctor was a "bad" practitioner. Clinical competence and the use of medical procedures, however, were not frequently used as criteria for evaluating a doctor, although the ability to carry out a thorough examination and make a referral to a hospital specialist were admired attributes. These results confirm evidence from other recent studies (Calnan et al. 1994) that patients, in assessing their family doctors, place great emphasis on the quality of their relationship with the doctor. The doctor's ability to listen, to be friendly and sympathetic, and to give time to the patient were qualities commonly referred to. It must, however, be emphasized that informants' assessments referred to their family doctors; criteria for assessing hospital doctors may be different because problems presented are more specific and the encounter between doctor and patient might be more routinized and structured (Calnan 1984).

Finally, what of the nature of the social relations with modern medicine and is there any evidence to show that some social groups are more "medicalized" than others? For example, has womens' greater experience of health care led them to be more or less critical of scientific medicine? Evidence from the second study showed that in relation to reproductive technology women were more accepting of hysterectomy than men were of vasectomy. This might reflect "real" differences between the procedures in that a comparison is not appropriate. However, it may also reflect, at least in part, the traditional gender division in responsibilities for contraception. Certainly, women seem to be more knowledgeable than men in this respect, which may reflect the different access to magazines and the greater use of contraceptive technology. However, in relation to the other technological procedures considered in the second study, there was no evidence to say that women were any less critical than men, indeed, with respect to tranquillizers for example, they appeared more so. Thus, while the medicalization theorists may be correct in asserting that women are more familiar with medical technology than their male counterparts, they are incorrect in assuming that this necessarily leads to a less critical stance (see Chs 9 and 10).

The two studies, however, portrayed different pictures in relation to social class and evaluation of modern scientific medicine. The argument offered for the evidence from the first study that working-class women were more sceptical than the middle-class women drew upon Abercrombie and his colleagues' (1988) ideas that the support of the working class for the dominant ideology was unnecessary as all that is required of them is to sell their labour to the market. However, the second study found the reverse was true, which suggests that the middle class may have been exposed to the demystification process previously discussed.

While social class position and gender may shape lay perceptions of modern medicine, evidence from other studies (Calnan & Williams 1992) using quantitative methods shows that age is also an important influence on lay views of modern medicine. Statistical evidence indicates a positive relationship between age and acceptance and satisfaction with medicine. A number of explanations have been put forward for this and some of the most common imply that either elderly people show greater deference or respect for medicine and doctors or they have lower expectations of health and health care. Alternatively, with their greater general experience of the procedures themselves, elderly people may have a better understanding of the uncertainties and recognize that as medicine becomes more successful and expands its jurisdiction the more difficult the problems it will have to solve.

In conclusion the evidence from these two studies shows that both men and women were ambivalent about the value of modern medicine and more specifically about certain drugs and medical procedures. Certainly they illustrate the limitations of the medicalization thesis. Indeed, as we have suggested, lay criticism appears to be the product of traditional beliefs and values as well as the broader processes of demystification and reflexivity that are currently taking place in late modernity: processes in which scientific knowledge and expertise is increasingly called into question and trust becomes active (Giddens 1991). However, these studies are limited not least in that they dealt with a heterogeneous group of people who varied in their direct experience of ill health and the specific procedures under investigation. Future research might therefore examine how far and in what way direct experience of a technological procedure and related health problems shapes lay evaluation (see subsequent chapter in this volume). Certainly, the lay populace seemed to be aware that there may be a difference between perceptions based on personal experience and more independent or general accounts.

References

Abercrombie, N., S. Hills, B. S. Turner 1988. *The dominant ideology thesis*. London: Allen & Unwin.

Calnan, M. 1984. Clinical uncertainty: is it a problem in the doctor–patient relationship? *Sociology of Health and Illness* **6**, 74–85.

Calnan, M. 1988. Lay evaluation of medicine. *International Journal of Health Services* **18**, 311–22.

Calnan, M. & S. Williams 1992. Images of scientific medicine. *Sociology of Health and Illness* **14**(2), 233–54.

Calnan, M., J. Coyle, S. Williams 1994. Changing perceptions of primary care. *European Journal of Public Health* **4**(2), 108–14.

Calnan, S. E. 1989. *Old people's perceptions of ageing and illness*. Unpublished MPhil thesis, Department of Social Psychology, University of Kent.

Cornwell, J. 1984. *Hard earned lives*. London: Tavistock.

Foucault, M. 1973. *The birth of the clinic: an archaeology of medical perceptions*. London: Tavistock.

Giddens, A. 1991. *Modernity and self identity*. Cambridge: Polity.

Habermas, J. 1971. *Towards a rational society*. London: Heinemann.

Haug, M. 1988. A re-examination of the hypothesis of physician deprofessionalisation. *Milbank Memorial Fund Quarterly* **66**(Supplement 2), 48–56.

Illich, I. 1975. *Medical nemesis: the expropriation of health care*. London: Calder & Boyar.

Karpf, A. 1988. *Doctoring the media*. London: Routledge.

Larson, M. 1978. *The rise of professionalism. A sociological analysis*. Los Angeles, California: University of California Press.

Parsons, T. 1951. *The social system*. London: Routledge & Kegan Paul.

Turner, B. S. 1984. *The body and society*. Oxford: Blackwell.

Waitzkin, H. 1979. Medicine, super structure and micro politics. *Social Science and Medicine* **13**(1), 601–19.

Part II
Medicines and drugs

Chapter 3

Lay views of drugs and medicines: orthodox and unorthodox accounts

Nicky Britten

Introduction

Compared with the extensive literature on lay beliefs about illness, the literature on lay views of drugs and medicines is sparse and is chiefly concerned with adherence to prescribed medication. However, before this literature can be summarized, two key definitional issues need to be resolved. First, from a medical perspective, the terms "medicine" and "drug" are often used interchangeably, yet from the lay perspective, there is evidence that the two words can have very different connotations. For example, several writers have drawn attention to the fact that, for some people, "medicines" are perceived as familiar and safe, while "drugs" are perceived as dangerous (Stimson 1974, Jones 1979, Helman 1981). In this chapter, however, unless otherwise stated, the two words will be used synonymously. Secondly, the frame of reference of this chapter includes all prescription and over the counter drugs but excludes drugs of abuse and illegal drugs. As the two categories cannot in fact be clearly separated, it is better to say that this chapter is concerned with drugs taken in the context of the treatment and prevention of illness rather than recreational or illegal usage.

Although many studies have been disease or drug specific, ideas about medicines have not been closely linked to ideas about illness. Much of the research has been concerned to show how ideas about medicines influence consumption of prescribed medicines. For example, Donovan & Blake (1992) in an interview-based study of people with suspected inflammatory arthropathy, showed how perceptions of risks and benefits affected adherence. Conrad (1985) examined the meanings of medication in the everyday lives of people with epilepsy, and showed that "non-compliance" was a way of asserting control over the disease. A few studies have shifted their focus from adherence to the social context of medicine taking. For example, Cooperstock & Lennard (1979) have written about the use of tranquillizers as a way of maintaining social roles, and Helman (1981) drew attention to the function of benzodiazepines in managing relationships with other people. The most detailed work is probably that of Fallsberg (1991) who described the conceptions of medicines held by a group of 90 people in Sweden on long-term treatment for hypertension, asthma and chronic pain.

The literature describes three main criteria by which lay people evaluate drugs and medicines: (i) efficacy; (ii) comparison with other therapies; and (iii) whether or not they are manufactured. Although there is evidence of faith in the efficacy of medicines (Conrad 1985, Clinthorne et al. 1986, Calnan 1988), this is often qualified. Several studies report the belief that drugs lose their effectiveness if taken over a long period of time (Donovan & Blake 1992) or that one may become "immune" to drugs that are taken too often (Stimson 1974, Fallsberg 1991). There are also concerns about side-effects (Morgan & Watkins 1988). In contrast to other therapies, there is evidence that people may prefer home remedies to drugs (Povar et al. 1984) or that in some contexts people may prefer to experience symptoms rather than take drugs (Gabe & Lipshitz-Phillips 1982). Some people may prefer traditional remedies (Morgan & Watkins 1988) or alternative medicine such as homeopathy or acupuncture (Power 1991). Lastly there is a concern about the perceived "unnaturalness" of manufactured medicines and drugs. For example, Coulter (1985) reported that women interviewed about their attitudes to the contraceptive pill switched from the pill because it was "unnatural", choosing instead sterilization, intrauterine devices or other mechanical means of contraception.

There is little evidence that people are becoming critical and challenging about drugs and medicines, although studies have not focused on this aspect of medicine taking. A crucial question here concerns whether or not people evaluate medicines and doctors separately. On the one hand, van der Geest & Whyte claim that medicines are metonyms, meaning that the medicine represents the doctor and in some ways can be considered part of the person:

> The medicine is an extension of the doctor. There is, as it were, a dose of the "doctor" in the medicine . . . The medicine stands for a less tangible experience of which it was a part, as the seashell serves as a memento for the beach one has known as a child (van der Geest & Whyte 1989).

On the other hand, doctors, medicines and doctors' prescribing habits could, in theory at least, all be subjected to separate evaluation. Although studies of lay health beliefs have distinguished "public" from "private" accounts (Cornwell 1984, see below), the same has not been done for lay beliefs about drugs and medicines. It is not known, therefore, which of the ideas referred to above are thought to have medical legitimation and which are not. In order to address these questions, this chapter applies Cornwell's theory of public and private accounts to lay views of drugs and medicines. However, for reasons given below, Cornwell's terminology will not be used in this chapter. Instead of referring to public and private accounts, this chapter will describe "orthodox" and "unorthodox" accounts respectively.

The data presented in this chapter are derived from a qualitative study conducted in London in 1991. Semi-structured interviews were conducted with 30 adult patients (21 attenders and 9 non-attenders) from two general practices. The sample consisted of 11 women and 19 men ranging in age from the early twenties to the seventies. The majority were white, there being only one middle eastern and two black interviewees. Nine people were registered with an inner city practice in a deprived area of London and 21 were registered with a suburban practice in an affluent area. The social class background of the sample is therefore mixed, although this was not formally measured on an individual basis. Questions asked in the interview covered response to minor illness, past and present medicine taking, expectations for prescriptions and opinions about doctors' prescribing habits, cashing of prescriptions and experiences of side-effects. The methods have been described more fully elsewhere (Britten 1994).

"Orthodox" and "unorthodox" accounts

Cornwell defined medicalization as the process through which people come to lose faith in their own knowledge and information, and in their own powers of judgement (Cornwell 1984). The term "medicalization" implies a relationship between two worlds which are different and separate from each other: the world of lay people and of commonsense health beliefs, and the world of medicine and of applied science. Cornwell argued that medicalization is one instance of rationalization (Habermas 1971). This is the process whereby social life is transformed, traditional legitimations being replaced by modern legitimations. The former are normative and involve values and beliefs, and the latter are scientific and technical, derived from analytic or empirical knowledge. This view of medicalization states that the dominant tendency in contemporary western culture is towards modern scientific and technical forms of legitimation, but does not imply that the process will necessarily take place everywhere and in all social groups, at the same pace or at the same time (see Ch. 1).

During an ethnographic study of working-class people in Bethnal Green in London, Cornwell found that medical and lay concepts of health and illness were related, but that the medical view dominated. Interviewees used both commonsense concepts of health and illness that had obvious connections with their own moral philosophy, and medical concepts or concepts they believed to be medical in origin. They also put forward commonsense concepts of health and illness that incorporated medical concepts and theories. It was less a matter of switching between two sets of concepts than of their commonsense beliefs reflecting and embodying the perspectives developed by experts. On the basis of these findings, Cornwell distinguished between two types of account: public and private. Public accounts were given in response to formal or direct questioning, and drew attention to ideas and values respondents believed were likely to win "public" approval. They described aspects of experiences, ideas and values that people believed were acceptable to doctors and compatible with a medical point of view. They were concerned with the moral aspects of illness, with the attribution of responsibility, and with acceptability and legitimacy. In contrast, private accounts were given when people were telling stories, and sprang directly from personal experience. Private accounts of illness were concerned with the context of illness, and with practical constraints and material issues. No legitimation beyond the respondent or a close confidante was sought. However, the difference between public and private accounts did not simply correspond to a difference between medical and lay concepts. Public accounts contained both, and switched between them, depending on the form of legitimation that was most applicable in that context. Nor was it the case that private accounts stood outside the medicalization process altogether, but the moral problem of allocating responsibility for illness was largely irrelevant and there was no attempt to claim medical authority when putting forward private aetiological theories. Public accounts of doctors were complimentary and deferential, and it was only in private accounts that people made critical remarks.

Cornwell's research was not especially concerned with ideas about medicines and treatment. However, her analysis can be used to make certain predictions about the ways in which drugs and medicines might be discussed in public and private accounts. Public accounts were concerned with the moral status of illness: Cornwell's respondents did not want to be accused of malingering but neither did they want to be labelled as sick. She argued that the most conclusive proof of the reality of an illness was a medical diagnosis. The issuing of a prescription by a doctor is a visible sign of the medical diagnosis, and thus one would not expect public accounts on the subject of drugs to be overly concerned with the reality of any condition for which treatment was prescribed. To be given a prescription is to have won the moral argument about the reality of the illness. The other side of this moral imperative in Cornwell's research was that people did not like to be perceived as having poor health, and described themselves as healthy even when they had major illnesses. Thus, whereas someone who has been given a prescription has won the moral argument about the reality of the illness, they nonetheless have to deal with the fact of being labelled a "sick" person. Therefore it might be expected that private accounts would reveal some dislike of drug taking.

The interviews that I conducted were classified using Cornwell's criteria. At the outset, it was not assumed that such a classification would in fact be possible. After all, Cornwell's research was based on a detailed ethnographic study lasting months, during which her informants were interviewed several times and came to feel that the research was a fact of their lives as well as hers. The private accounts took some time to elicit, and it could not be assumed that a study based on one-off interviews would contain any private accounts at all. Additionally, in my study it was not possible to determine whether each interviewee did in fact have both a public and a private account, nor to conclude that one or other type of account came closer to what people "really" believed. It therefore seemed appropriate to use a different terminology that did not imply that there were layers of reality such that behind each public account lay a private account. Given the emphasis on the presence or absence of medical legitimation, it was decided to label the two types of account in this study as "orthodox" and "unorthodox". In the process of classification, Cornwell's criteria were refined. Four specific criteria derived from Cornwell's description of public accounts were used to classify orthodox accounts, and five specific criteria derived from her description of private accounts defined the unorthodox accounts. These criteria will now be described.

The first criterion for orthodox accounts was that of medical legitimation. Interviewees cited medical opinion in justification of all or most of their actions or beliefs. They also said that they had faith in their doctor and did what their doctor told them to do. Some pointed out the folly of ignoring the doctor's advice and others said that they had accepted their doctor's recommendation even if they had reservations. Some interviewees giving orthodox accounts seemed anxious not to criticize doctors, although this does not mean that orthodox accounts were devoid of criticism. Others provided justifications for doctors' potentially culpable behaviour. The second criterion for orthodox accounts was a concern with the legitimacy of illness, although this was not a major issue, perhaps for the reason already given. The third criterion was the absence of self-legitimation, in contrast to the unorthodox accounts (this issue is discussed more fully below). These three criteria all related to the content of the interviews, while the fourth criterion related to the interview process itself. There were cues in some of the interviews that established the status of the interview as an orthodox account. One interviewee asked me several times if he was giving me the answers I required. Another interviewee made reference to her GP records, implying that I could check the truth of what she was telling me. This woman, who was interviewed in the surgery, also referred to the tape recorder:

> I mean you're the only person I've ever told that to, I mean now probably about nine million other people . . . (D29: orthodox).

Sometimes I had noted at the time that I felt I was not being given the whole story. These processual cues were never the only criterion for classifying an interview as an orthodox account, but reinforced the other criteria. The two main criteria were the presence of medical legitimation and absence of self-legitimation.

Two of the criteria for classifying an interview as an unorthodox account were exactly the opposite of those used to classify an interview as an orthodox account. The first criterion was self-legitimation. Some interviewees made this explicit by saying things like "I believe" or "I have a belief". They also spoke of their own "philosophy and the moral ideas of taking chemicals" (D5: unorthodox) and "the role and the fight that I have to live without medicine" (D7: unorthodox). Self-legitimation could be less explicit, when interviewees gave their own opinions or devised their own ways of taking medicines, without seeking or citing medical legitimation. Occasionally views were legitimated by non-medical significant others, and this is included in self-legitimation. The second criterion for unorthodox accounts was the absence of medical legitimation, established by what was missing from the interviews, in contrast to what was present in the orthodox accounts. However some interviewees acknowledged that their account contradicted the medical model, by referring to their own "disobedience". Others overtly rejected medical dominance or said that they did not believe doctors. In some cases medical legitimation was sought but not obtained, for example when interviewees had experienced side-effects and wanted confirmation from their doctors. The third criterion was the stated view that there was no single medical model. Several interviewees said that different doctors had different views, undermining the notion of a monolithic medical model. The fourth criterion was the appeal to "unorthodox" legitimation, usually alternative medicine, but also including the media and psychology books. As with the orthodox accounts, the final criterion was to do with the process of the interview itself. Several interviewees said that the interview was confidential or "off the record", or explicitly asked me not to tell their doctor what they had said. One man made this clear when I asked him what he did with prescriptions:

I'm very glad that this interview is confidential. I have been known to get prescriptions from a doctor and because of the role and the fight that I have to live without medicine I very often put that in my pocket and never actually cash it (D7: unorthodox).

Of these five criteria the first two, self-legitimation and the absence of medical legitimation, were the most important.

Using these criteria, seven interviews were immediately classified as orthodox and eleven as unorthodox accounts. Of the remaining twelve, seven needed re-examination and five were unusable (three of the latter had not been recorded, one was inaudible, and the last was the transcript of a confused elderly man whose account defied classification). The seven transcripts that needed re-examination raised difficulties that helped to clarify the boundary between orthodox and unorthodox accounts. Two of these were precarious interviews in the sense that they were borderline, and the interviewee had to make obvious efforts to prevent them crossing the boundary. One was a woman giving an orthodox account, into which crept themes typical of the unorthodox accounts, which she then "repaired". For example when asked if she had ever failed to cash a prescription, she said that she had a prescription (apparently for a non-hormone treatment of menopausal symptoms) in her bag at the moment.

NB: And when you get given a prescription by the doctor do you always cash it?

No, well yes, I mean to say no. I've got one in the my bag now which is the most unusual thing because it's the first prescription I've ever got that I've kept . . . but that is about the only time I've ever hung on to a prescription. Every other time I have just cashed it in and got it (D9: orthodox).

She obviously did not want to present herself as a "non-casher" of prescriptions, whereas those giving unorthodox accounts said openly that they sometimes failed to cash prescriptions. Later on she expressed surprise that doctors were "pushing" hormone replacement therapy but repaired this criticism by saying that "obviously it's become more of the thing now than it was a few years ago". Again, those giving unorthodox accounts frequently complained of overprescribing doctors.

The other precarious account was an unorthodox account in which the interviewee hesitantly attempted to provide medical legitimation for his behaviour. Having said that he "knocked the dosage off slowly myself" (D13: unorthodox) of antibiotics prescribed for acne, he then said that he went to the doctor and told him what he had done, and the doctor had accepted this. He put forward the view that over-use of antibiotics leads to "immunity" and said that his doctor "might" have told him this.

The five remaining transcripts that needed re-examining were all difficult to classify because the interviewees' unorthodox accounts had been shared with their doctors. In the end they were all classified as unorthodox accounts because interviewees were not seeking medical legitimation for their views. They made it clear that their views were their own, and that they were pleased to find that their doctors agreed with them.

The final result of this classificatory exercise was that there were eight orthodox accounts, seventeen unorthodox accounts, and five unusable interviews. That there were so many unorthodox accounts may be a result of the fact that, unlike Cornwell's sample of working-class people in Bethnal Green, the present sample contained a number of middle-class people. As a consequence the social distance between the interviewees and the medical profession, or between the interviewees and myself, was much less than in Cornwell's research. Indeed, some of the interviewees spoke about doctors as their social equals, or had family or friends who were doctors.

Data on past and present medicine taking and on interviewees' ages were tabulated against the types of accounts given. People giving orthodox accounts were more likely than those giving unorthodox accounts to be currently taking long-term medication for chronic illnesses such as asthma or ongoing problems such as acne. Of the eight people giving orthodox accounts, four were on long-term medication compared with four of the seventeen giving unorthodox accounts. All the interviewees had taken antibiotics at some time in the past. Those giving orthodox accounts were likely to be older: half of them were of pensionable age compared with only two of the seventeen giving unorthodox accounts. However not all long-term medication was attributable to the elderly, as two of the four people of pensionable age were not currently taking any drugs.

Having established the basis on which the interviews were classified, the content of the orthodox and unorthodox accounts will now be described.

"Orthodox" accounts of medicines and drugs

Cornwell's public accounts contained both medical and lay concepts, and respondents switched between the two. Similarly the orthodox accounts of medicines and drugs in this study contained some elements also present in unorthodox accounts. However, the converse was not true. The orthodox accounts will be presented under four main headings: correct behaviour, own use of medicines, doctors' prescribing habits, and potential criticisms of doctors.

Correct behaviour

In various ways interviewees giving orthodox accounts presented themselves as behaving correctly. They all said that they always cashed prescriptions, some adding that it was daft not to. Most of them said that they always took the medicine in the way that they were supposed to, and some pointed out the folly of ignoring the doctor's advice. One woman who was interviewed in the surgery and gave a very obviously orthodox account said:

> Yes I do because quite frankly I can't see the point of coming to the doctor if you're not going to use what he suggests you, you know, that is a total waste of time (D29: orthodox).

Some were willing to accept the doctor's recommendation that they take a prescribed medication even if they had doubts, for example about its potential addictiveness. In various ways they expressed deference to their doctors, by being complimentary about them, expressing faith in them, saying that they did not disobey them, and taking care not to criticize them. Some said that patients were not qualified to tell doctors what to do. Several were very conscious of the doctor's time, saying that they did not waste it nor rush to the doctor at the first sign of illness, and were aware of the "hungry horde" in the waiting room when they did consult.

Own use of medicines

Half of those giving orthodox accounts were on long-term treatment for chronic illnesses. Medicine taking was a routine part of their daily lives that did not evoke much comment unless something went wrong. The following story was given by an elderly woman (interviewed in the presence of her husband) who was on long-term anti-hypertensive therapy and who also used analgesics and an inhaler every day:

> One Christmas, we always remember this story, we had people sleeping in our bedroom so we had to make do with a bed in here and our tablets are in there, mine's my side of the bed and [husband's] is his side, and so we left them in there, got up made a cup of tea. That must have been our normal what seven o'clock . . . about ten o'clock I thought God I do feel ill. We still hadn't thought about the tablets and without me knowing [husband] wasn't feeling good . . . all of a sudden about ten o'clock it clicked, he hadn't taken his tablets and I hadn't taken mine so we were three

hours late taking them and I was very surprised that it would affect us as much as it did . . . we take them regular every morning . . . with our first cup of tea (D10: orthodox).

Some people knew what medicines they wanted for certain conditions and said that they asked, or told, their doctors to prescribe what they wanted. Others expressed disapproval of people who asked for prescriptions because they felt that patients did not know enough to make decisions about treatment.

There were some themes in orthodox accounts that were also present in unorthodox accounts. Several interviewees gave examples of medicines that had been ineffective, or said that they had stopped taking medicines after experiencing side-effects. Some had managed to wean themselves off addictive drugs such as benzodiazepines. An elderly widow who had been taking Temazepam for years had managed to reduce the dosage:

Well I've been on tranquillizers for years and I need them. And I've cut them down enormously in strength but I do sleep badly. And I believe if you really give them up it can be dangerous if you stop dead . . . it would bother me if my doctor cut me off completely . . . she's quite pleased with how far I've got with her (D15: orthodox).

Another view common to both types of accounts was the feeling that one should be able to "sort one's illness out" oneself without resorting to medication if at all possible. The idea that over-use of antibiotics would lead to some kind of "immunity", rendering them ineffective when really needed, was common in the unorthodox accounts but was also present in the orthodox accounts.

Doctors' prescribing habits

When asked about doctors' prescribing habits those giving orthodox accounts usually said that doctors' prescribing was "about right". What this meant was that interviewees got what they needed, one elderly woman saying that she always got a prescription if she wanted one. Some explicitly said that their doctor never prescribed too much or that they had not been given prescriptions to get rid of them. The following quotation is taken from a professional woman in her thirties who had been taking antidepressants for some time:

I never feel when I am in there that, my goodness, they are trying to get my bottom off the seat, never, in fact when I'm in there I've almost forgotten that there is a hungry horde outside waiting to come and see them. So I have never felt that I have been palmed off with a prescription and felt unhappy that isn't exactly what I was expecting (D6: orthodox).

If there were complaints from this group, they were about under-prescribing. There were several stories of patients not being given prescriptions when they thought they needed them. The woman just quoted described an incident when she felt a prescription was warranted:

he actually prescribed nothing, and there I am propped up with this bronchial thing thinking you know am I going to survive the night which is actually what [boyfriend] thought at the time, I think he thought I was going to peg out, he prescribed a Dr Johnson's inhaler bottle thing which flabbergasted me . . . (D6: orthodox).

However, complaints about underprescribing were not confined to ortho-dox accounts.

Potential criticisms of doctors

Although those giving orthodox accounts were less critical of doctors than those giving unorthodox accounts, a few criticisms were nonetheless voiced. Some potential criticisms were not presented as such, or were defused. This was particularly true of side-effects. The elderly widow already quoted was given something to help her sleep while she was cutting down on the Temazepam:

it gave me a stomach upset, so after about four days I stopped. And I mentioned that to her, I said I had to stop so and so I was feeling ill, and she said yes that is a side-effect you know (D15: orthodox).

Others who experienced side-effects did not report them to their doctors but neither did they use the experience to criticize doctors. Another elderly woman had used ointment that had burned her skin:

Then he gave me another lot [of ointment] when he came last Monday, and I put that on and I had to put the cream on as well, after. And after I didn't know whether I had to wash it off and put the cream on, or put the cream on top of it. Then it started burning. I did it again. I felt oh I suppose it's me, you know. And I had to keep putting cold flannels on me. I couldn't stand it . . . So I left it off. I mean I haven't told them – I haven't seen him. I've just sorted myself out.

NB: And you don't feel like going back to the doctor and saying, look this ointment burnt me?

No, no.

NB: Why wouldn't you like to go to the doctor?

Well, he can only give me this, can't he? (D1: orthodox).

Another view was that side-effects were inevitable and that there was no such thing as a "safe" drug. This was put forward by a retired medical journalist, not currently taking any medication himself, who was very critical of other journalists' "hysterical" stories:

If you're going to find material, chemicals that do things, that cause changes in a body then if they're going to be any good at all with the illness or whatever is wrong with you they are going to have side-effects, by definition . . . You know there's still a lot of people who believe you can have a safe drug . . . there's no such thing in the world (D19: orthodox).

There were some concerns expressed about medicines in this group but they were muted. The woman who was reducing her dose of Temazepam had some fears:

I've sometimes said to the doctor "what do you think about this new thing that older women are taking?" and, you see I love to have all the benefits of modern medicine but I'm very scared about side-effects or anything else (D15: orthodox).

When criticisms were made, they tended to be about "other doctors" than the interviewee's own doctor, or about doctors in the past. Some acknowledged that other people criticized doctors but distanced themselves from these criticisms. Direct criticism tended to be about the organization of the practice (such as waiting times) rather than the doctor personally.

"Unorthodox" accounts of medicines and drugs

Although the orthodox accounts of medicines and drugs contained elements also present in unorthodox accounts (for example stories of people stopping medication that was disagreeing with them) the converse was not true. All the themes discussed below were exclusive to unorthodox accounts.

Aversion to medicines

The people giving unorthodox accounts had their own ideas about medicines that were almost entirely negative. Medicines were variously described as artificial, chemical and unnatural. This is because they are manufactured and are not natural in the sense that flowers grow naturally. A young man in his twenties who took intermittent medication for hay fever said:

> I try to take them as and when needed, you try not to use them much. I don't know why. I mean I'm not really worried about using them . . . it's not necessarily a natural substance you're putting inside you (D13: unorthodox).

A young woman also in her twenties who took alternative medicines such as homeopathic and Bach Flower remedies explained why she preferred these to more orthodox treatments:

> It's the chemicals I suppose . . . I just don't like artificial things . . . [natural remedies] are not chemically made, like flowers are naturally grown things. I prefer to take those than factory made chemicals (D2: unorthodox).

However, as Calnan & Williams (1992) note, the category "natural" is far from self-evident, and merits further investigation. One of the interviewees did in fact comment on the definition of this category. An engineer, he was discussing the evolution of the techniques of "fringe medicine":

> how do you define synthetics, you've taken a bunch of flowers and stewing it in a pot, synthesizing a chemical . . . you're cooking it so you're synthesizing it effectively, or do you go to some super chemist who gives you a designer drug? I mean three handfuls of buttercups and four of nettles, is that the same as, I don't know, three atoms of this and four atoms of that in the final result. One's practical, one's theoretical (D23: unorthodox).

Pharmaceuticals were also described as being "foreign to the body", as an "alien force", and as "intruding on the body". The underlying theme behind all these statements was that pharmaceuticals were harmful to the body, the most extreme assertion of this position being that all medicines are carcinogenic:

> I have a belief whether I am right or wrong that all medicines to an extent are carcinogenic. It's like everything else if you take enough of it and overdose over a long period of time you are always prone to perhaps . . . advancing the nature of things like cancer . . . (D7: unorthodox).

This statement was made by an articulate middle-aged man who was not taking any medication at the time of the interview. Various mechanisms were described by which pharmaceuticals manifested this damage. They were described as lowering the body's resistance to infection and disease. For some this was to do with reducing the body's ability to combat infection naturally by preventing the immune system from working. For others this was seen to result from the fact that pharmaceuticals actually damaged the immune system. A man in his thirties, not taking any medication at the time of the interview, had a lot to say about antibiotics:

> I've got . . . a lot of ideas that antibiotics aren't good for my body, that they actually reduce my ability to combat infection naturally . . . my belief is that antibiotics do stop the functions or the antibodies, your own antibodies, the immune system performing . . . I think antibiotics do actually harm the body in some way . . . maybe it knocks out the . . . body's ability to create the necessary chemicals or white corpuscles or whatever they are to deal with the situation. It maybe hinders the situation (D5: unorthodox).

These views were echoed by another man in his late forties who was also not taking any medication at the time:

> the adverse publicity about the attack on people's, the effect on the immune system . . . the understanding may not be correct that antibiotics really don't correct the virus, they may get rid of other symptoms, problems, but the virus in the end has to be defeated by the body's system and so it seems that natural ways can be, you know, just as effective as an antibiotic (D11: unorthodox).

As the above quote makes clear, another aspect of the mechanism was that pharmaceuticals were seen as dealing with the symptoms and not the cause. Even if the symptoms were successfully cured, the underlying problem would not have been dealt with and thus the treatment would only be partial. Since pills would not alter the external situation, the situation would still have to be faced when the pills were stopped. This was explained by the engineer quoted above:

> if you've got something wrong with you which produces certain symptoms, if you can't cure the problem you just cure the symptoms. OK you've still got something wrong with you but you feel OK which is effectively what you do with headaches. You're not curing the headache as such . . . you're just dulling the senses that are telling you you've got a headache . . . not actually getting to the root of the problem which is actually giving you the headache (D23: unorthodox).

Pharmaceuticals were perceived as offering uniform treatments, in other words not being tailored to the needs of individuals. As each individual experiences symptoms in a slightly different way, uniform prescriptions were not seen as being necessarily effective for any particular individual. The man who spoke at length about antibiotics said:

> actually I don't see a lot of medicines as being effective to the symptoms as each symptom is slightly different for every person, having a general uniform prescription or drug . . . to suit everybody is not going to do the same for everybody . . . it's like trying to match up two pieces of a jigsaw, they are not going to fit for everybody (D5: unorthodox).

Two interviewees, both of whose somewhat negative views were quoted above, gave more balanced assessments in the sense that they acknowledged the positive contribution that pharmaceutical medicines had made:

> one tends to rubbish the whole western system and yet when you look at what it has done it's fantastic, so you know I'm actually quite a supporter of it (D11: unorthodox).

> I do think medicines are good. I do think there is a place. It is not that I disagree with medicines but I feel that they are abused (D2: unorthodox).

Preference for not taking drugs

Many of those giving unorthodox accounts said that they preferred not to take medicines if it could be avoided. A man in his mid forties, who was not taking painkillers recently prescribed for joint pain because of side-effects, explained:

> it's not worrying me that much that I think I ought to take medication because I tend not to like taking medication if I can avoid it.
>
> NB: Can you say a bit more about that?
>
> Yes I think nature has its own way of mending things in many cases . . . I'm always slightly wary of drugs of any sort really, I mean other than paracetamol . . . if I don't feel I need to take them, I won't take them (D24: unorthodox).

The young man who did not take his hay fever medication as prescribed said:

> I think why take something if you don't necessarily need it . . . I'm not frightened of taking them at all but if I don't need them I won't use them (D13: unorthodox).

Related concerns were about long-term or stronger medication. A building labourer who had been prescribed long-term medication for chest pain the day before the interview, was reluctant to start taking them even though the pain interfered with his ability to work:

> I don't want to be stuck with them for the rest of my life (D17: unorthodox).

The man who thought that all medicines were potentially carcinogenic was particularly concerned with long-term medication:

> To give you the bottom line, short term I'm not worried, long-term medication I would be worried (D7: unorthodox).

The strength of the medication was also an issue for some:

> if I suddenly . . . became a diabetic for instance I would need insulin and I think if I could possibly avoid taking particularly strong medicines and strong drugs I would hope to avoid it (D5: unorthodox).

This interviewee also made explicit the links between medicines and sickness, and his own unwillingness to be labelled:

> I suppose what I feel mostly about medicines and prescribed medicines is that they are for sick people and if I can avoid being sick then I can avoid medicines and not have to have them in my body (D5: unorthodox).

Some said that they did not like having medicines around the house, because they were tempting, either for themselves or for their children. Others said that they did not need prescriptions from the doctor to prove that they were ill, or that they did not expect miracle prescriptions to solve their problems immediately. Less negative statements were made by those who said that they used to have trust in medication, or those who had taken medication in spite of their reservations, and had been helped as a result. Several interviewees who were averse to taking medicines did describe the circumstances in which they would be prepared to take something. Symptom severity, particularly pain and high temperatures, was an important triggering factor. Interference with the ability to perform at work was another, and less frequently mentioned was the interference with having fun. A few of those giving unorthodox accounts said that they would take antibiotics for infections or if the doctor recommended it.

One of the main features of the orthodox accounts was the emphasis on correct behaviour, in particular the cashing of prescriptions. In contrast, those giving unorthodox accounts often gave examples of not cashing prescriptions. Usually this behaviour was not discussed with the doctor, but occasionally interviewees said that they had been given explicit permission by their doctors not to cash prescriptions. An airline manager who had caught an infection abroad and had been given antibiotics in hospital was given another prescription for the same drug by his GP:

> I had a follow up meeting with Dr X at the surgery and he said "oh look I'll give you a prescription in case you ever need one again", I'm probably committing a terrible indiscretion, I don't know whether they are supposed to issue prescriptions on that basis, but he said "look if you're going away again, pick up a packet of Flagyl or whatever" . . . and I've still got the prescription (D21: unorthodox).

Some of those giving unorthodox accounts said that they always cashed prescriptions, because they only went to the doctor when things had become serious enough for them to want medication, and they wanted to take something immediately. One man who had said earlier in the interview that he was "deeply suspicious of anything" explained why he cashed prescriptions straight away:

> if it's got that critical that I've gone to the doctor, then I want to stick something in me quickly to get rid of whatever it is that's upsetting me . . . if I feel bad enough to go to the doctor then I want something done quickly (D23: unorthodox).

The man who thought all medicines potentially carcinogenic explained his attitude towards adherence:

> Yes, I'm an absolute stickler for that, although on the one side I say I don't take any medicine, once I do actually take them I'm an absolute stickler for the number of times a day and the times it's prescribed (D7: unorthodox).

Criticisms of doctors

Most comments about doctors in the unorthodox accounts were negative, and the most common criticism was about overprescribing. Interviewees complained that it was hard to leave the consulting room without a prescription, although some acknowledged the pressures on doctors that made such behaviour convenient for them. A non-attender who had little personal experience of the health centre but whose wife and children had received many prescriptions made a typical comment:

> My own opinion is that I think they probably prescribe too much. I think you're lucky to come away from the doctor without a prescription for some pills (D25: unorthodox).

A young mother who was very concerned about the amount of antibiotics prescribed for her children acknowledged some of the reasons why doctors might overprescribe:

> I know that in the past frustrated doctors have given bottles of totally innocuous liquids to "old dears" to sort of make them feel better (D30: unorthodox),

as did other interviewees including a man who hardly ever went to the doctor:

It's probably quite understandable for the doctor when he sees Mrs B for the fifteenth time that year with some ridiculous ache or pain and he just gives her something to get rid of her . . . that's probably cost effective from his point of view to see her out of the way (D21: unorthodox).

Another criticism, linked to overprescribing, was the failure to place the prescription in context:

Well, apart from that they prescribe too much . . . they don't always place the prescription within the context of the whole experience . . . explain what the prescription's doing and give you the feeling as a patient that they understand the sort of life that you lead and how the prescription is part of that life (D22: unorthodox).

The consequences of overprescribing in terms of drug wastage were described by one man who had experienced unpleasant side-effects:

I think they prescribe too much. I'm going now not by my own experience but my wife's experience. I remember on one occasion she had something or other and she needed to take paracetamol. I've got enough paracetamol in the house to feed an army, you know, great boxes and boxes of them . . . in the past certainly I think they prescribed too much and you end up throwing them, half of them, away (D12: unorthodox).

Linked to this, some interviewees had been very pleased when their doctors had not prescribed and had explained that a prescription was not necessary. One man had moved from a practice where he felt the doctors prescribed too readily to a practice whose approach he was much happier with:

Though I was encouraged recently . . . the doctor explained to [son] about the undesirability of taking too much in the way of antibiotics (D22: unorthodox).

Others commented more generally about the overuse of medicines without attributing it to doctors:

there is so much forced at you nowadays and medication is so easily available . . . even the supermarket where you do the food shopping . . . it's totally unnecessary 90, 95 per cent of it (D14: unorthodox).

Two men commented on the status of doctors in less than deferential ways. One, an engineer, said that doctors were like mechanics, working on a trial and error basis. The other, who had experienced side-effects and who also identified the pharmacist as an important source of information, was critical of medical dominance:

> there is still this big authority thing in the medical profession in that the views of the patients aren't sought, that they aren't consulted in the first place, that we have to respect what the doctor tells you and the lingering feeling that the doctor knows best . . . frankly I see the thing I referred to earlier about the failing to clarify side-effects of drugs as part of the same sort of mystique (D22: unorthodox).

Discussion

This discussion will address the three main themes of this book: the nature of lay perspectives of drugs and medicines; the criteria used by lay people in evaluating drugs and medicines; and the extent to which people are coming to question or challenge their doctors on this topic. In exploring the nature of lay perspectives, this chapter has distinguished between orthodox and unorthodox accounts, chiefly on the basis of the presence or absence of medical legitimation. Yet how clearly separated are these two types of account? In other words, was there any evidence of ambivalence? Another key question here concerns how far a lack of reference to medical legitimation in unorthodox accounts was due to the taken-for-granted nature of medical knowledge and its superiority. While some of the themes described in the orthodox accounts were also present in the unorthodox accounts, the converse was not true. The themes common to both types of account were not presented as medically legitimate in the unorthodox accounts. The interviews that were hard to classify were the ones in which interviewees' own ideas had been brought into the consultation, but these ideas were self-legitimated and not medically legitimated. In other words, none of the ideas described in unorthodox accounts were presented as medically legitimated, and there was little evidence of ambivalence. Interviewees who gave unorthodox accounts were not asked if their own views were superior to those of their doctors, although some of them pointed out that their views contradicted medical orthodoxy. No conclusions can be drawn therefore about the perceived superiority of orthodox or unorthodox views.

This study is based on single interviews, and these and other questions about the status of orthodox and unorthodox accounts can only be answered by longitudinal ethnographic research. For example, do orthodox and unorthodox accounts correspond to Cornwell's public and private accounts respectively (Cornwell 1984)? Do most people have both an orthodox and an unorthodox view of medicines, and does one type of account more closely represent what people "really" believe? Perhaps each type of account is partial, so that a more rounded picture can only be drawn by considering both types together. What is also unclear is whether unorthodox accounts correspond to what Habermas (1971) referred to as traditional legitimations. In other words, it is not clear whether or not they have historical roots. Certainly Calnan & Williams (1992) suggest that these kinds of beliefs are, at least in part, a product of traditional values.

The criteria used by interviewees to evaluate drugs and medicines confirmed those reported in other studies, but there were marked differences between those giving orthodox and unorthodox accounts. In fact those giving orthodox accounts showed little evidence of making any evaluation, instead displaying a taken-for-granted view of drugs and medicines. There was an implicit, if not always explicit, belief in the efficacy of medicines in the orthodox accounts, whereas potentially harmful effects were emphasized in the unorthodox accounts. Both groups mentioned side-effects and their consequences for adherence, but those giving unorthodox accounts were more critical of doctors as a result. Both groups also compared medicines with other kinds of therapy, although this theme was stronger in the unorthodox accounts. However, the main difference between the two types of account was that while those giving orthodox accounts talked about medicines in a taken-for-granted fashion, those giving unorthodox accounts showed what can only be described as an aversion to medicines. Reference to the perceived "unnatural" and "damaging" properties of medicines, previously reported in other studies, was only made in the unorthodox accounts. What this study suggests, therefore, is that the themes of "unnaturalness" and "harm" are not perceived to have medical legitimation.

It is possible that these ideas are linked to the rejection of science and the scientific endeavour (see Ch. 1). In this study, medicines perceived as "unnatural" were contrasted first with "natural" experiences, in other words untreated symptoms or illness, and secondly with "natural" remedies, such as plants or herbs. In both cases, science-based treatment was avoided. However, this topic is in need of further exploration, as perceptions of what is "natural" or "unnatural" are far from obvious. For example, in Coulter's (1985) study, it was not clear why sterilization was perceived as more natural than the oral contraceptive pill.

In considering the evidence from this study about lay criteria for evaluating drugs and medicines, there is little to suggest that people evaluate doctors and medicines separately. Although the present study cannot answer this question definitively, it would seem that criticisms of medicines and criticisms of doctors (especially their prescribing habits) tended to go hand in hand. If this is so, then it may be that patients who are uncritical of their medicines are those who do not want to criticize their doctors. Van der Geest & Whyte's (1989) claim that the medicine is a metonym for the doctor seems to be supported by the data presented in this chapter.

The last question is whether the data presented in this chapter provide any evidence that interviewees were questioning or challenging their doctors. Anyone familiar with the discourse about prescriptions is struck with the apparent contradiction between lay and medical views. A common theme in medical discourse is the demanding patient who insists on being given a prescription particularly for minor self-limiting illnesses such as coughs and colds (Bradley 1994). On the other hand, the overprescribing doctor is often criticized by patients (Calnan 1988). It can only be concluded that doctor–patient communication on this subject is poor: a conclusion entirely supported by Tuckett et al.'s (1985) research. They showed that there is little elucidation of patients' ideas in most medical consultations. In their research, doctors and patients did not manage to achieve a dialogue and so did not share or exchange ideas to any great degree. Patients often limited the chance of dialogue and in this sense did not make it easy for their doctors. Tuckett and colleagues suggested that the reason for patients' silence was that when they did behave more openly, the consultation often became tense. After the consultation, patients often explained their silence by saying that they were frightened of the doctor's response, felt hurried or thought that their doctor might think less well of them. Other studies have similarly documented patients' passivity in medical consultations (Boreham & Gibson 1978).

One explanation for this passivity and lack of communication is that patients are voicing orthodox accounts within the consultation, and keeping their unorthodox accounts to themselves. This seems very likely given the overriding concern with medical legitimation and acceptability in the former. Patients are probably well aware that their unorthodox accounts lack medical legitimacy. The orthodox accounts of drugs and medicines emphasized correct behaviour in the form of cashing of prescriptions and the taking of medicines as directed, often in a very taken-for-granted fashion. If this is the view that doctors are presented with, then they may well perceive that patients want prescriptions most of the time. From the patient's perspective, however, their unorthodox agenda, being unvoiced, will not have been attended to. It will appear that the doctor is merely concerned with giving prescriptions. The unorthodox accounts of drugs and medicines were almost entirely negative and revealed strong aversions to medicines and medicine taking. If such views are not aired in the consultation, then any advice or treatment offered by the doctor is unlikely to take account of them.

The majority of interviewees in this study did not think that their doctors knew what they thought about drugs and medicines, confirming the results of Tuckett et al.'s (1985) research. However, a small number of those giving unorthodox accounts had communicated their ideas to their doctors, or at least had found a doctor whose ideas coincided with their own. These were the very interviews that were difficult to classify, precisely because the "unorthodox" agenda had been brought into the consultation. In the words of the insurance salesman who was concerned about the effects of drugs on his driving, when asked if his doctor knew what he thought about medicines:

> I think she does, yes . . . I think she's pretty switched on . . . she always knows or seems to know that, well he's not always looking for tablets, so I don't have to give him some (D16: unorthodox).

Another way in which patients can bring "unorthodox" ideas into the consultation, not reported in this study, is to show magazine or newspaper cuttings to the doctor. Although this was not an issue explicitly explored in the interviews, the data suggest that the media may play some kind of intermediary or mediatory role between orthodox and unorthodox accounts (see Chs 1 and 4). In the unorthodox accounts, the media were sometimes used to legitimate negative views of medicines, while negative media coverage was clearly a problem for some of those giving orthodox accounts:

> Well they're always on about tranquillizers being . . . so bad for you, and they've got a thing called Tranx which is supposed to stop people, but I watched it, it was a programme and I thought a lot of the women were very hysterical about it, as if taking any kind of pills was life threatening (D15: orthodox).

Perhaps the media are partly responsible for creating unorthodox accounts, or perhaps they help to bring unorthodox views into the public domain. Is there a dynamic process by which unorthodox views gradually become orthodox, and do orthodox accounts contain criticisms of the medical profession which have been legitimated by the media? Such questions are beyond the scope of the present study, although Gabe and colleagues (1991) do suggest that the media perform a mediating role of a slightly different kind. These issues are further discussed in Chapter 4.

Orthodox and unorthodox accounts may also be characterized as corresponding to passive and active patients. In orthodox accounts interviewees were deferential to doctors and willing to be guided by them. In unorthodox accounts, interviewees had their own views and made their own decisions. Patients presenting their orthodox persona to the doctor may appear passive and willing acceptors of medical dominance, but once the consultation is over, the "patient" regains the possibility of active control. This suggests that for those who fail to bring their own ideas into the consultation, any questioning or challenging of medical legitimation will occur outside the consulting room. The form that such challenge is likely to take, on the basis of the data presented in this chapter, is criticism of doctors' prescribing habits and non-adherence to prescribed medication.

The difference between active and passive patients has implications for Cornwell's (1984) definition of medicalization, which, as we have seen, is the process through which people come to lose faith in their own knowledge and information, and in their own powers of judgement. Although people may realize that their unorthodox accounts do not have medical legitimation, this is not the same thing as losing faith in their own judgement. Medical dominance may suppress articulation of unorthodox views within the consultation, but subsequent behaviour may be determined by people's own views rather than by what is thought to be medically legitimate. In particular, aversion to medicines is likely to result in non-adherence to prescribed medicine. All medicine taking outside institutional care is self-medication in the sense that the individual decides whether or not to take the drug, when, where, and in what quantities. Whereas there is a vast body of medical research into "non-compliance" that has confirmed over and over again that a substantial proportion of patients do not take their medication as prescribed, it has failed to explain *why* this happens (Meichenbaum & Turk 1987). It seems very likely that this behaviour, so problematic from a medical perspective, is informed by people's unorthodox views. Research conducted from a medical perspective, therefore, is unlikely to reveal the reasons for "non-compliant" behaviour if patients realize that their views are not medically legitimate. The "problem" of "non-compliance" is the failure of medicalization to extend beyond the consulting room into the spheres of everyday life where people take their medicines. Hence, the challenge to medical dominance may occur not in the public but in the private realm, in the guise of non-adherence to prescribed medication.

References

Boreham, P. & D. Gibson 1978. The informative process in private medical consultations: a preliminary investigation. *Social Science and Medicine* **12**, 409–16.

Bradley, C. 1994. Learning to say no: an exercise in learning to decline inappropriate prescription requests. *Education for General Practice* **5**, 112–19.

Britten, N. 1994. Patients' ideas about medicines: a qualitative study in a general practice population. *British Journal of General Practice* **44**, 465–8.

Calnan, M. 1988. Lay evaluation of medicine and medical practice: report of a pilot study. *International Journal of Health Services* **18**, 311–22.

Calnan, M. & S. Williams 1992. Images of scientific medicine. *Sociology of Health and Illness* **14**, 233–54.

Clinthorne, J. K., I. H. Cisin, M. B. Balter, G. D. Mellinger, E. H. Uhlenhuth 1986. Changes in popular attitudes and beliefs about tranquillizers. *Archives of General Psychiatry* **43**, 527–32.

Conrad, P. 1985. The meaning of medications: another look at compliance. *Social Science and Medicine* **20**, 29–37.

Cooperstock, R. & H. L. Lennard 1979. Some social meanings of tranquillizer use. *Sociology of Health and Illness* **1**, 331–47.

Cornwell, J. 1984. *Hard–earned lives: accounts of health and illness from East London*. London: Tavistock.

Coulter, A. 1985. Decision-making and the pill: the consumer's view. *The British Journal of Family Planning* **11**, 98–103.

Donovan, J. L. & D. R. Blake 1992. Patient non-compliance: deviance or reasoned decision-making? *Social Science and Medicine* **34**, 507–13.

Fallsberg, M. 1991. *Reflections on medicines and medication: a qualitative analysis among people on long-term drug regimens*. Linköping, Sweden: Linköping University.

Gabe, J. & S. Lipshitz-Phillips 1982. Evil necessity? The meaning of benzodiazepine use for women patients from one general practice. *Sociology of Health and Illness* **4**, 201–9.

Gabe, J., U. Gustaffson, M. Bury 1991. Mediating illness: newspaper coverage of tranquilliser dependence. *Sociology of Health and Illness* **13**, 332–53.

Habermas, J. 1971. *Toward a rational society: student protest, science, & politics*. London: Heinemann.

Helman, C. G. 1981. "Tonic", "fuel" and "food": social and symbolic aspects of the long-term use of psychotropic drugs. *Social Science and Medicine* **15B**, 521–33.

Jones, D. R. 1979. Drugs and prescribing: what the patient thinks. *Journal of the Royal College of General Practitioners* **29**, 417–19.

Meichenbaum, D. & D. C. Turk 1987. *Facilitating treatment adherence: a practitioners' guidebook*. New York: Plenum.

Morgan, M. & C. J. Watkins 1988. Managing hypertension: beliefs and responses to medication among cultural groups. *Sociology of Health and Illness* **10**, 561–78.

Povar, G. J., M. Mantell, L. A. Morris 1984. Patients' therapeutic preferences in an ambulatory care setting. *American Journal of Public Health* **74**, 1395–7.

Power, R. 1991. People choosing their health care: an initial analysis of some Mass Observation Data from the Spring 1984 Directive on Health Services and Sickness. Paper presented to the British Sociological Association Annual Conference, Manchester.

REFERENCES

Stimson, G. V. 1974. Obeying doctor's orders: a view from the other side. *Social Science and Medicine* **8**, 97–104.

Tuckett, D., M. Boulton, C. Olson, A. Williams 1985. *Meetings between experts: an approach to sharing ideas in medical consultations*. London: Tavistock.

van der Geest, S. & S. R. Whyte 1989. The charm of medicines: metaphors and metonyms. *Medical Anthropology Quarterly* **3**, 345–67.

Chapter 4
Risking tranquillizer use: cultural and lay dimensions

Jonathan Gabe & Michael Bury

Introduction

Concern about risk has been increasingly prominent in academic and public debates in recent times. Where there was once optimism about scientific progress, and an acceptance of the authority of experts and expertise, now, apparently, risk reigns supreme. Modern societies, it is held, are increasingly coterminous with risk, arising from "manufactured uncertainty" that is associated with the need for ever increasing "reflexivity" (Giddens 1991, 1994, Beck 1992a,b). Now, everyday life comprises knowledgeable people assimilating large amounts of technical information about risk, much of it potentially contradictory or unclear. Such information circulates at an ever faster rate, issued from "abstract systems" and produced by increasing numbers of experts, who may be "lay people" except in specialized areas (Giddens 1991, 1994, Beck, 1992a,b). In a "destabilized" and "runaway world" the landmarks of a more certain era give way to "de-skilling" and "re-skilling" by turns.

In this setting lay people, themselves, can take a leading role in challenging authoritative knowledge, as exemplified by campaigns around environmental health risks such as toxic waste (Brown 1992, Williams & Popay 1994) and perceived risks arising from managing serious mental illness in the community. The coverage of such campaigns in the media influence people's awareness of such risks (Short 1984) and may play an important role in encouraging them to challenge expert authority.

Perhaps these examples also help explain the recent upsurge in academic writing on risk, namely their elective affinity with expressed concerns about the impact of a volatile and threatening social environment as well as that of risks produced by technology and science, especially, in the context of our discussion, medical science. However, there are reasons to be cautious about the current academic debate on risk. One of the main problems is that it proceeds by painting a highly generalized picture. Giddens (1991), for example, argues, that "manufactured risk" has now taken over from "natural risk", but does not examine closely how "natural risks" in the past were perceived and managed, and thus how characteristic or indexical current preoccupations are. As a result, it is difficult to judge how important the putative causes and effects of living with risk today are, and how different the current situation is from previous periods (modern society being loosely referred to, as "post-traditional social order" in Giddens' most recent work (1994: 5)).

Moreover, empirical evidence on the variable impact of risk on everyday life is noticeable by its absence. This is particularly apparent in the health field where the little work that has been undertaken has generally focused on health risk behaviours such as drug injecting (McKeganey & Barnard 1992), unprotected sex (Holland et al. 1992), road behaviour (Bellaby 1990), reproductive risks concerning childbirth (Handwerker 1994) or the transmission of a genetic disease (Parsons & Atkinson 1992).

As can be seen little consideration has been given by sociologists to lay perceptions of the risks of medical technology, especially in its most widespread form, namely medication. The aim of this chapter is to try to help rectify this situation by looking in some detail at the available evidence about lay evaluations and responses to risk in one area of medical treatment – the use of benzodiazepine tranquillizers and hypnotics to treat anxiety and insomnia. Although less widely prescribed than in their hey day during the late 1970s, 15 million scripts for these drugs were dispensed in 1993 (DoH 1995) and there are still thought to be 1.2 million people taking them on a long-term basis of a year or more (Ashton & Golding 1989).

We begin with the way in which people's risk perceptions of benzodiazepines, like other medical treatments, are culturally framed especially by the mass media. We then go on to review evidence about the use of these drugs in everyday settings, focusing in turn on lay perceptions of risk, managing the risks of tranquillizer consumption and the social risks involved in the use of these drugs.

The cultural framing of risk

It is commonly acknowledged that the mass media are the major vehicle for communicating health risks (Nelkin 1989). While people also seek risk information from other sources such as general practitioners (OHE 1994) or personal contacts (Douglas 1985), television and the press provide a critical "frame" or context within which the public and private shaping of health risks can be interpreted and understood (Nelkin 1991).

The considerable media coverage given to the risks of taking benzodiazepine tranquillizers over the last 30 years provides an important example of the way in which the media frames perceptions of risk. When they were first prescribed to patients in the early 1960s the media gave the benzodiazepines a generally enthusiastic welcome. For instance, in 1960, in the US, *Time* magazine talked about Librium, the first of the benzodiazepine family, as a new drug heralding a new era, and claimed that it came close to "producing pure relief from strain without drowsiness or dulling of mental processes" (*Time* 1960).

As this new generation of tranquillizers became more and more popular, however, their therapeutic value ceased to be newsworthy. Instead more critical coverage developed from the mid 1970s onwards (Cohen 1983), drawing on the comments of a small but growing number of professional and lay critics, and ending the brief celebration of an apparent breakthrough in the effective treatment of at least one area of "minor" psychiatric disorders.

The reasons for this change in emphasis are difficult to explain in causal terms, particularly as there was a relative paucity of large-scale scientific evidence about side-effects at this time. The media, however, keyed into and helped create what they perceived to be a shift in "public mood" with regard to drug therapies, towards a moral rather than scientific set of concerns (Conrad 1994). Articulating an approach to tranquillizer use involving a mixture of moral approbation, sympathy and a challenging tone, the media have reproduced here what Morley (1992) suggests was also developing in other areas – a dominant media style, in which public policy issues can be tackled by recourse to commonsense judgements. Indeed Morley maintains that the construction of "commonsense judgements" has been the defining ideological characteristic of media treatment of such issues. With respect to the benzodiazepines, public concern about the large-scale and widening use of these drugs in the 1970s meant that the line between their use for people suffering from debilitating illness and those with milder symptoms may have become effaced (an issue currently reverberating around another therapeutic drug – the anti-depressant, Prozac (Kramer 1993)). But instead of examining the complexities of these changes in health patterns and medical practice the media mounted a series of challenges against the drugs as a whole.

In one of the first media attacks (Cohen 1983), in 1975, *Vogue* warned its US readers of "Danger ahead! Valium – the pill you love can turn on you". Quoting a US psychiatrist the magazine asserted that taking Valium could result in a far worse addiction than heroin, morphine or meperidine. Such claims were soon endorsed in the USA in books written by journalists (Hughes & Brewin 1979), ex-users (Gordon 1979) and medical consumer groups (Public Citizen Health Research Group 1982). All saw tranquillizers as exemplars of the American "pill-popping" way of life (Montagne 1991).

Similar claims about the risk of these drugs' "addictive" potential also began to appear in the British media around the beginning of the 1980s, picking up statements of experts or ex-users and the media coverage emanating from the USA. For instance, the *Observer* (1980a,b) devoted 1¼ broadsheet pages over two weeks to "The dangers of tranquillity". Using case studies of users and interview material with British and American medical experts and health care professionals, it described the "physical dependence" on Valium estimated to be experienced by up to 5 per cent of users and offered advice about how to minimize the risks involved in taking the drug. Subsequently, the *Standard* (London) (1981) ran an article based on the publication of Diane Harpwood's (fictitious) diary of a house wife Valium "junkie", under the headline "Why the happy pills have had their day". The article described the drudgery and frustration of the housewife portrayed in the diary and the way in which reliance on Valium perpetuated this state of affairs. This "addiction" theme was also developed in a page long article in the tabloid newspaper, the *Daily Mirror* (1982). Under the headline "The dangers of the happiness pill" it reported the release in the USA of the film, *I'm dancing as fast as I can*, based on the life of the American television producer Barbara Gordon who had become a "victim of the Valium trap".

Benzodiazepine dependence continued to attract media attention for the rest of the decade. Between 1983 and 1985 the British Broadcasting Corporation (BBC) television consumer magazine programme *That's life* considered the issue on at least four occasions. Drawing on viewers' letters, it presented powerful images of users, mainly women, being taken over by the drugs, experiencing startling results of withdrawal and being caught in a spiral of dependence (Bury & Gabe 1990). The programme's viewing figures reached 10 million people and it was reported that it generated an unusually large postbag. One thousand letters were received after the first programme, and 40,000 people responded to the invitation after the programme in May 1984 to write to MIND for a leaflet on tranquillizers (Lacey & Woodward 1985). The *That's life* programmes married together "commonsense" views of the topic with a powerful appeal to the domestic and almost suburban context in which television has become increasingly embedded in the last 20 years (Silverstone 1994).

Subsequently, two other major television programmes in Britain focused on tranquillizers and transmitted dramatic images of "addicted" patients. In 1987 the BBC current affairs programme, *Brass tacks*, dealt with the issue on two occasions watched by 2.5 million viewers each time. And the following year Central Television's *The Cook report* devoted one of its prime time slots to the controversy surrounding a particular benzodiazepine,

Ativan, with viewing figures of 6 million. In order to convey the nature of the content of this coverage, it is worth noting that in both of the above programmes the early sequences either described or showed an individual patient hooked on these drugs. On the first *Brass tacks* programme the opening sequence was of a man drawing up a "fix" of an injectable tranquillizer. In *The Cook report* graphic representations of drugs showering down from the top of the screen were created in order to press home the message of dependence, reinforcing a story of one woman user's attempt to withdraw (Gabe & Bury 1991).

While the gender of users was implicit but unacknowledged in these programmes it did become the focus of attention in a number of "how to" books, written by British journalists and academics in the mid 1980s following feminist critiques of tranquillizer prescribing as a means of medicalizing women's distress. Melville (1984) and Curran & Golombok (1985), for example, both produced accessible paperbacks for sale on bookstalls that dealt with the gender imbalance in use, the "facts" of addiction and withdrawal and the availability of alternatives, ranging from counselling to yoga.

The continuing interest in "addicted" users was also apparent in press coverage in the late 1980s. An analysis of 62 stories concerning the personal experience of tranquillizer use reported in the local and national UK press in 1988 found that ordinary users, most of whom were women, were presented as innocent victims of the drug, succumbing to "evil" through no fault of their own and embarking on a metaphorical journey to "hell and back" (Gabe et al. 1991). However, when women reported that they had tried to withdraw from using the drugs, they appeared more as active consumers, aware of the effects of tranquillizers and capable of deciding to stop and embark on a return journey, as it were, back to a normal life. In this way media coverage has framed the ambiguities in the use of licit mood altering drugs, by rehearsing the moral dimensions of an otherwise health-related behaviour (Conrad 1994). The form that this coverage has taken has changed "addiction" from being associated with deviant groups to being a risk that can be encountered in everyday life.

Media coverage of the risks of taking tranquillizers has continued into the 1990s. In the UK press attention shifted to the issue of litigation embarked on by "tranquillizer addicts" and their lawyers. Journalists reported the progress of the case under headlines such as "Judge gives claim deadline for tranquilliser addiction" (*Independent* 1991) and, "Deadlines set for addiction case claims" (*Daily Telegraph* 1991). When the major test case finally collapsed in 1994, after legal aid was withdrawn from Ativan claimants, headlines referred to the "Sad story of the happy pills" and described how the legal system appeared unable to cope with a "group compensation claim for tranquilliser addiction" (*Guardian* 1994).

As far as television is concerned, particular attention has been given in recent coverage to the alleged risks of taking the benzodiazepine sleeping tablet Halcion. In the UK the BBC current affairs programme *Panorama* (1991) highlighted the admitted under-reporting of adverse reactions to the drug, including paranoia, through interviews with prisoners and ex-prisoners who had been involved in a clinical trial in the USA to establish the drug's efficacy and safety (Gabe & Bury 1994). The story was subsequently picked up by the American media and, in particular, by the investigative television news programme *60 minutes* (CBS 1991). In Britain, the *Panorama* coverage was found to be libellous in one of the longest and most costly libel cases to be heard in British courts in modern times (Hall 1994).

From the above account one can see that the media have found the risks of unwanted side-effects of benzodiazepines newsworthy for a considerable period of time. Like other such stories, particular attention has been paid to accounts of individual users, reflecting the journalistic imperative for dramatization and personalization (Gabe et al. 1991). A preference for the language of "addiction", with its connotations of illicit drug use, alongside images of users, mainly women, as passive victims, are likely to have grabbed the readers'/viewers' attention and helped provide a public, and especially moral framework within which tranquillizer use could be interpreted and understood. As with the transmission of other risk information, however, people are most likely to have assimilated and interpreted these messages in line with prior beliefs and personal experience (Nelkin 1989). It is to this critical question of lay perceptions of risk that we therefore now turn.

Perceiving risk in using benzodiazepines

While media coverage of the risks involved in taking tranquillizers provides an important context within which to situate their use, risk perception needs to be seen as an active process, shaped by personal beliefs, social circumstances and experience. In the case of benzodiazepines we can see how these factors have interacted over time to provide a changing and complex picture of lay risk perceptions.

In one of the first studies of users' views Linn & Davis (1971) reported the survey findings of a community sample of 100, middle-aged, Californian women. The results revealed at that time a high degree of satisfaction with the effectiveness of psychotropic drugs being taken. Apparently, 59 per cent of those taking these drugs were very satisfied and a further 29 per cent were classified as "somewhat satisfied".

A more detailed picture was provided by a national survey of 2,552 US adults aged 18 to 74 conducted in 1970–71 (Manheimer et al. 1973). This study revealed that most of those asked (74 per cent) believed that tranquillizers were effective, and condoned their use when asked to make a judgement about a concrete situation in which a person's ability to function was severely impaired. At the same time, however, reservations were expressed about their propriety, with two-fifths claiming that taking tranquillizers was a sign of weakness and four-fifths agreeing with the statement that it is better to use willpower to solve problems than use tranquillizers. It is apparent from such findings that the moral dimension found in media coverage is paralleled in lay people's views. A similar level of concern was revealed when respondents were asked about the drugs' safety. These attitudes were also related to people's wider value orientations and their personal drug use. Those seeing tranquillizer use as a sign of moral weakness also scored highly in terms of other values commonly associated with the Protestant work ethic, regardless of age, income or gender. Users of tranquillizers were also more favourably disposed towards the drug than were non-users.

A follow up to the 1970 study was undertaken in 1979 (Clinthorne et al. 1986). Based on interviews with 3,161 US adults, this study revealed that beliefs about the presumed negative effects of tranquillizers on health had become more widespread among men and women, and users as well as non-users of these medications. For instance, more than eight out of ten people in 1979 agreed that tranquillizers often have bad side-effects (compared with just over seven out of ten in 1970) and 90 per cent agreed with the statement that long-term use of tranquillizers may cause real physical harm (compared with 80 per cent in 1970). Respondents were also less willing than in 1970 to condone the use of tranquillizers in situations involving moderate impairment but were as willing as before to condone use in situations in which individuals were seriously incapacitated by emotional distress. These findings were explained in terms of an increase in the perception of risks associated with use in the late 1970s, interacting with, and thus influenced by, media coverage. It was argued, however, that risk perceptions continued to be offset by the benefits of treatment where emotional distress was seriously debilitating.

More recent evidence of lay risk perceptions with regard to tranquillizers comes from small-scale qualitative studies undertaken in the UK. These paint a complex picture of the perceived risks of tranquillizer use at a time of heightened public concern and media coverage. In one such study, Gabe & Thorogood (1986) undertook semi-structured interviews about the meaning of tranquillizers with 60 middle-aged women from East London. When asked what they felt about taking these drugs a range of opinions were expressed. Some stated that they were concerned about the danger of becoming dependent on or "addicted" to tranquillizers and felt that they might be harming their body or mind by ingesting such "unnatural" substances. Others said they felt these drugs were helpful in that they offered them "peace of mind". Yet others expressed both views, illustrating a common but often unrecognized feature of the ability of lay thought to hold conflicting or contradictory elements (Young 1976). Overall a quarter emphasized only the unwanted risks and a tenth only the benefits: the remaining two-thirds expressed mixed views. From this evidence it seems clear that taking tranquillizers crosses boundaries between warrantable behaviour (treatment for illness) and moral culpability (not "coping" and being reliant on the "crutches" of a drug) (Gabe & Bury 1988).

In order to illustrate the nature of these views, it is worth quoting from some of the interview data from the Gabe and Thorogood study. The ambivalence is well captured, for example, in the following remarks, where one woman stated:

> I've never liked taking pills unnecessarily unless it was really that I couldn't stand it, then I would take them. But otherwise I don't like [them]. I take Librium but without it I wouldn't be able to go out . . . If I have a backache or something or anything I try not to take pills. I don't really like taking pills.

And another user commented:

> When I take Valium my mind goes blank. I don't worry about anything. It will all sort itself out. It just sort of puts my mind at ease . . .

Later on, however, the same respondent admitted:

> I'm not really one for taking tablets. I think once you get hooked on these Valium you've had it you know. You really are hooked on them.

Not surprisingly, women who were long-term users – that is those who said they had used tranquillizers consistently over the previous ten years[1] – were most likely to express positive feelings, whereas the non-users – those who said they had not received a prescription for the drug over the previous decade – were the least likely to do so.

Negative sentiments were often reinforced by knowledge of friends' or relatives' experiences of taking tranquillizers, or by adverse coverage in the mass media. For example, a non-user drew on knowledge of a relative's experience when she stated:

I think it can be a habit forming thing. My sister-in-law takes a lot of Valium and tablets and all sorts of things. But I think you can tell yourself you can't do without them. You know if she hasn't got a Valium to go to bed at night, she can't go to sleep. You know, she's got to have that! I'm sure she could go to sleep if she wanted. Only she's got into the habit of taking them. I wouldn't like that. I hate to be dependent on anything really. I'm really an independent person I suppose.

Similar ideas about the risks of "addiction" and moral character were referred to by a long-term user when discussing television as a source of information about tranquillizers.

There was one [television programme] that particularly stuck out in my mind and may be that subconsciously had an effect on me . . . where people have become hooked on them. But obviously they were taking much more than me. And the way they described, you know, the um – I mean one woman I think almost had a nervous breakdown because . . . when she stopped taking them. And I thought, "Well, that isn't going to happen to me" you know.

In sum, perceptions of risk in taking benzodiazepines in this study were mediated by the experience of personal usage and by the knowledge of others' experiences, relayed first hand or through the media. In the case of "first-hand knowledge" it is also clear that lay evaluation occurs within a moral framework, involving family relationships and segments of specific communities. Similar evidence of risk perceptions has been provided in a related study by Gabe & Lipshitz-Phillips (1982, 1984) and by Calnan & Williams (1992) in their study of modern medicine and medical practice, which included questions about tranquillizers (see Ch.2). These findings are also in line with evidence on the perception of risk in other areas of health, notably that on risk from heart disease (Davison et al. 1991) where respondents were aware of official messages about risk but also drew on lay knowledge of illness in family and community settings in evaluating them.

At the same time that the studies of tranquillizer use discussed above were being conducted, Helman (1981) also reported evidence of lay risk perception in this area, though it emerged as a less significant issue. In Helman's study, 50 older (average age 60+) and mainly female, long-term benzodiazepine users were interviewed in North London. While Helman found that around a third of his sample emphasized the benefits of taking these substances, claiming that they had resulted in some improvement in

82

their mental state, a larger number (40 per cent) denied any subjective change after taking the medication. Among these respondents, doubt was frequently expressed as to whether the tablets had any pharmacological effect and their impact was described as "probably psychological". According to Helman this interpretation may have been a way of reducing the drug's symbolic significance as a drug of dependence and helping the respondents regain a sense of autonomy.

Even so, a fifth of the sample in the study reported unwanted side-effects, including nightmares, depression and impotence, and four-fifths recognized that they were taking "a drug" even though most of them were against taking "drugs" in general. Apparently they qualified their moral disapproval by pointing out that their use of benzodiazepines was an unfortunate but necessary evil in the face of a lack of perceived alternatives. Such moral disapproval of "drugs" in general was said to reflect the negative connotations attached to "drug taking", involving, as noted, a loss of control and a sufficiently altered state of consciousness that the person may feel that she can no longer function in daily life. The question of control has also been found to be central to lay ideas about health in other areas (Crawford 1984).

Helman also noted that friendship and family networks played an important role in providing his respondents with ideas and information about tranquillizers. In his study, however, it appears that the users' social network generally approved of taking these drugs with many of them taking the same drug themselves. Awareness of taking the same prescribed medicine was said to create a bond between members of the network, as illustrated by the following remarks:

All my friends are on Valium.

All the widows are taking something.

Nearly everyone I know (is taking Valium).

This contrasts with the finding of Gabe et al. and may reflect, in part, the rapidly changing cultural climate with regard to benzodiazepines and other prescribed medicines in the early 1980s. Paradoxically, it may mean that the controversy surrounding tranquillizer dependence has led to a greater awareness of the availability and use of these drugs and a more sympathetic view of users. It may also illustrate differences in risk perception between different age groups, with older users being less risk conscious, though further work is needed on variations in perceptions of risk across age and gender groups. What does seem to be clear, however, is that media coverage and lay perceptions now include images of a more active patient where the everyday management of risk becomes normalized.

Management rather than the desire for minimization has increasingly characterized responses to risk in recent years. It is therefore to this issue of everyday management that we now turn in a little more detail.

Managing the risks of tranquillizer use

The relationship between the cultural shaping and perception of risk, on the one hand, and health behaviours on the other, is always likely to be a complicated matter. Though we cannot presume to "read off" behaviour from stated views, it seems clear in the case of tranquillizer dependence that the ambivalence expressed in respondents' accounts does influence the practical management of the drugs in daily settings.

In the study by Gabe & Thorogood (1986) the meaning that the respondents gave to their drug use appeared to be clearly related to their pattern of use. On the basis of their comments two kinds of "risk management" were identified. For some, benzodiazepines were used as a *life-line*; that is something that they needed to take regularly and depended on simply to keep going in the face of chronic, unresolved problems, and where risks of dependence might be viewed as less pressing than other problems. Others appeared to see the drug as a *standby*, to be kept in reserve and used occasionally to meet some short-lived crisis, hence keeping dependence at bay. Yet others seemed to draw on both kinds of usage. However, four-fifths of the women appeared to look upon their drug taking in only one way, with similar numbers seeing their tablets as a life-line or a standby.

These two approaches to tranquillizer use are illustrated in the following quotations, first as a life-line:

> My sleeping tablets I can't do without them at all. One every night. I can't get off them. I'm dependent on them for a sleep. I've got to have them.

And second as a standby:

> Sometimes, if I'm very worried, I have one. I don't take them regularly. I hate taking tablets anyway. But if I'm feeling very agitated and I've got to go somewhere, got to go out, then I take one and I find they calm me down.

These women's comments about the use of their drug are illustrative of common patterns found across the study group. Those who conceived of the drug as a life-line were most likely to be long-term users whereas those who conceived of it as a standby were generally short-term users;

with the latter meaning that the respondent had used the drug for a couple of weeks at a time and over a two-year period at most. Again, perception and management were closely related. Those who talked of relying on the drug as a life-line expressed mixed or positive views, with most choosing to voice the former; whereas those who used it only as a standby expressed mixed or negative views in equal numbers.

Helman (1981) has also developed a typology of tranquillizer users' relationship with their drugs, although the focus in his case was on the meaning of such usage, the degree of control over tranquillizers exercised by respondents, and their mode of action. In particular, tranquillizers in this study were regarded from an anthropological perspective as *tonic, fuel* or *food*. Patients who saw benzodiazepines as a *tonic* were said to express maximum control over their drug use, using it episodically, and emphasizing their own responsibility for use, rather than difficulties in their relationships. They also minimized the drug's pharmacological power in their comments. Those who saw their medication as a *fuel* managed a variable degree of control over it and said that it enabled them to function in conformity with familial and social expectations; whereas those who represented the drug as a *food* expressed little control over its use, and adopted a management style where they took it at fixed times and saw it as necessary for their sanity and the survival of their relationships.

The main difference between this typology and that of Gabe & Thorogood (1986) is that the users' management of their drugs is presented by Helman in more positive terms, with less emphasis on risk and more on drugs as nutritional substances. As a result of focusing on control and mode of action as the key dimensions, the typology fails, however, to take sufficient account of respondents' responses to risk perception and their consequence in everyday use.

From this viewpoint it can be argued that the lay management of the risk of dependence, and other unwanted side-effects, in tranquillizer use is not only a product of the meaning of the drug, but also of social context. This brings into the picture such factors as the availability of and involvement in paid work, the presence of active social support, and commitments to religious beliefs. Gabe & Thorogood (1986) highlighted the role of these resources in explaining different patterns of tranquillizer use among indigenous, white working-class women and their West Indian born black counterparts.[2] They noted that indigenous women reported using benzodiazepines more often and over a longer period than the West Indian women although they expressed a similar range of views about the risks of taking them. Where they differed was in terms of the availability of other resources. The black women were more likely than the white women to have a full-time job and to view such employment as enabling, perhaps reflecting their greater economic need and historical desire for financial independence (Stone 1983, Bryan et al. 1985). This may help explain why black women found it less necessary to resort to benzodiazepine use on a long-term basis.

The black women in Gabe & Thorogood's study were also more likely than the white women to have children living at home and to find their female children particularly supportive, offsetting, perhaps, the need to risk taking tranquillizers.

As one West Indian woman remarked about her daughter:

> When I turned 40 and I was pregnant I was really worried. I didn't think I could cope. But today she's such a helpful one in the family. Oh dear, she's my right hand. She's useful, obedient, everything.

Again this bond between black working-class mothers and their daughters is explainable historically in terms of the development of the West Indian family structure that has traditionally forced women to take the major, if not sole responsibility for the family's wellbeing (Standing 1981).

Finally, they found that the black women were far more likely than the white women to describe themselves as regular church goers and to state that their religious practices helped them to manage their daily lives. As one black respondent put it:

> Praying, now that's special. You got to do that, haven't you, as a telephone link to the master of all. I don't have to go to church to pray – I walk along and say a little prayer. Every day of my life I do that. It does help you get by. God is your friend and your father – he's always there – you know he's there. So if you've got something bothering you and if you don't want anyone to hear, like I don't want him [husband] to hear, I just whisper it to him and he hears, he knows . . . He is my best friend, my very best friend.

Such sentiments were most often expressed by those black women who were short-term users or non-users, suggesting that religion played a major part in reducing the likelihood of their becoming regular long-term users. These women's willingness to attach such significance to religion is, again, unsurprising given the historical importance of religion in the West Indies (Pearson 1981), especially for women (Foner 1978).

Gabe and Thorogood's study also revealed the lack of certain key resources that constrained white women who were long-term users to maintain this pattern of drug use, despite their awareness of the risks involved. The women involved not only had access to fewer resources than short-term users, but those to which they did have access were not experienced as sufficiently enabling to allow them to manage their lives without taking tranquillizers regularly. They were markedly less likely to have a full-time job and if they did they were more likely find it unfulfilling than other women in the study. They were also more likely to be divorced or not have children living at home with them, or to be living with family members who were not supportive, compared with other white women. And they were much more likely than these other women to state that they either lacked all opportunities for leisure or had few leisure options open to them. It was therefore concluded that white long-term tranquillizer users' access to and relationship with these three resources – paid work, children and partners, and leisure – combined to produce greater reliance on tranquillizers and overrode perceptions of negative risks.

This is not to suggest that even long-term tranquillizer users are totally constrained to continue taking their medications indefinitely, or that they are not influenced by perceptions of risk. The study by Gabe & Lipshitz-Phillips (1984), based in part on interviews with 39 middle-aged, female, long-term users, revealed that half of these users said they had managed to stop and most of these claimed that they had done so on their own initiative. They reported that they had been motivated to stop either because they feared they were becoming over-reliant on their tablets, because they were worried by the drug's physical side-effects or, more positively, because they no longer needed them. The latter view was explained by one woman in the following terms:

> I got sick of taking them [Valium]. I mean they weren't for my health, put it that way. They weren't there to make me physically better. They were there really only to put my mind out of action. And I didn't want that. So I just thought to myself "It's all in your mind, girl. Get rid of them pills and you'll be as right as rain" and I was.

Not surprisingly, those who used benzodiazepines as a standby were markedly more likely to have stopped taking them recently or in the past. Similar findings about long-term users' attempts at withdrawal and the motives behind such actions have been reported by Murray (1981) and King et al. (1990). Thus, as with perceptions of risk, practical management turns out to be more complex and socially patterned than is often recognized.

Having said this, there is one further aspect to the risks involved in taking tranquillizers that we need to consider, albeit briefly – what we here term "social risks".

Social risks and benefits

Although we have focused so far on the health risks involved in taking tranquillizers it is also necessary to consider whether there is any evidence of social risk. By this we mean two related issues; one, the risk of moral opprobrium and potential stigma resulting from being seen as a "drug user", and, two, the risk of being seen to be unable to cope without the use of tranquillizers, of "needing a crutch" to rely upon. Against this we are also interested in whether there are social benefits in taking tranquillizers that outweigh these social risks.

Helman's (1981) study, referred to earlier, suggests that some people taking benzodiazepines emphasize certain social benefits. For example, when asked about the supposed effects of the drug on their relationships, a quarter of the people in the study stressed the advantages for their social lives. For these people the impact was indirect; taking their medication enhanced their emotional state and that benefited other family members. Another 15 respondents, who did not report any social benefits from taking tranquillizers, did feel their relationships would suffer if their drug supply was halted. They said they would feel socially inadequate or "incomplete" without the drug and would only be returned to normal social functioning if their medication was obtainable again. This view was expressed particularly by elderly widows.

Such social benefits from taking tranquillizers are reflected in the following statements:

[Without it] I'd be miserable – take it out on the family.

[Without it] I'd be nasty, jumpy, not nice to live with.

[Without it] I couldn't help those I love.

[Without it] I'm morose – don't want to talk – withdrawn.

What was of particular note in Helman's study was that the risk of stigma did not loom large in benzodiazepine use. Most people said they had told others about taking these medications and some indicated that a shared knowledge of drug taking had created a "community of suffering", offsetting a wholly negative moral attitude towards the use of these drugs. Only nine patients reported moral disapproval from others for using benzodiazepines. The rest either experienced approval or a neutral response.

The evidence from a Canadian study by Cooperstock & Lennard (1979), however, places greater emphasis on the social risks of use. Fourteen group interviews with 68, mainly female and middle-aged, participants revealed that tranquillizers were often used to help women and men continue in stressful roles and that the women in particular were critical about being given a drug when what they felt was needed was a practical or material solution to their problems. Reliance on the drug was seen in socially negative terms, as the following female respondent demonstrates:

> I think the thing that upset me most about the way [tranquillizer] drugs were used with me was that in the early years when I was so obviously unhappy with what was happening in my life, the solution to the doctors was so obviously a drug solution. And I had to push everybody I knew, except my psychiatrist who supported me all the way, that the solution for me was going to be really to quite radically change my life and not to make me comfortable with the life I was in.

In addition, the sample included a small number of people who had been prescribed tranquillizers as an adjunctive therapy for a chronic physical illness. These informants all expressed frustration and anger about how the drug had been used to mask their emotions and thus prevent them from rejecting the "sick role" that was often imposed on them by the nature of their illness and their family members. Using tranquillizers added to their social problems rather than relieving them.

For example, one informant who was suffering from lupus erythematosus, said:

> they were using drugs to cover up my true feelings, because with as much anger and hate or anything I had in me I never voiced my anger to my husband or to his family or anyone whom it was obviously directed at. And consequently they knew I was upset, which I was with just cause. So they gave me Valium and Serax and everything. But that did not solve the problem at all because they didn't even know I was angry with them. Then one day I blurted it out and they came and grabbed me and said, "Why didn't you tell us? We kept doing this to you because you never said anything. You left yourself wide open." Which was very true . . .

The limited evidence about the social risks involved in taking benzodiazepines is therefore mixed. For some it seems that the social benefits outweigh the risks, but this is not universally so. Some people, particularly women and the chronically ill seem to take the opposite view. For them the fact that they were taking tranquillizers added to the negative reactions of others. Though the evidence is somewhat contradictory, we have drawn attention to it here as a dimension of risk, as the impact of perceptions and management of tranquillizer use on social relationships have largely been neglected.

Conclusion

In this chapter we have highlighted lay people's risk perceptions of benzodiazepine tranquillizers, their management and attendant social risks, and the way in which such risks have been framed by the media's abiding interest in these drugs. It is clear from our account that people have become more ambivalent about these drugs, as the media have increasingly emphasized the risks of "addiction" if benzodiazepines are used for any period of time. However, despite widespread disquiet and media criticism, it is also clear that such ambivalence includes a measure of acceptance of tranquillizers and their role in everyday life.

The more preponderant negative aspects of lay people's heightened awareness of the risks involved in taking these drugs may be seen as part of a more pervasive "anti-drug" culture (Gabe & Lipshitz-Phillips 1982; see also Ch. 2). Fears about ingesting unnatural substances are now widespread, fuelled by the negative publicity surrounding a range of medicines from contraceptives to anti-rheumatics (Gabe & Bury 1991), the increasing popularity of alternative medicines (Saks 1994) and the zeal of campaigning groups such as anti-vivisectionists (Elston 1994). These concerns in turn resonate with a shift towards a more conservative (or "neo-liberal") moral order, based on personal responsibility, abstinence and self-reliance (Hall 1983), but also on autonomy and personal freedom. It is against this backdrop that people's views about the risks of taking tranquillizers need to be understood. People are having to fashion responses on a moral terrain with few landmarks, yet are also asked to display considerable reflexiveness in doing so (Beck 1992a, Giddens 1994). Difficult though this social pathway is, the evidence reviewed here shows just how far people are actively able to hold clear views and adopt workable strategies in meeting life's contingencies.

By the same token, the evidence presented here would seem to challenge the relevance of the medicalization thesis as it applies to tranquillizers, at least at the micro-level.[3] While commentators have argued that the main effect of prescribing these drugs has been to encourage patients, especially female patients, to become dependent on them and discourage them from any attempt to handle their own lives (Koumjian 1981, Ettorre 1985, 1992), the picture appears more complex. Rather than finding all tranquillizer users suffering from dependence and passivity, we have discussed evidence of a range of responses. These were seen to be based on people's personal and social experience, their knowledge of the effects of the drugs and the availability of a range of material and socio-cultural resources, which might help them get by without recourse to tranquillizers.

In sum, users of these drugs are best seen as active agents, weighing the risks of use against the need for drug therapy to help them with their personal problems, on the basis of available knowledge and existing resources. The question of resources also brings into focus the importance of social structure and social context in the management of risk. Autonomy and reflexiveness may be important cultural motifs, but our evidence suggests that structural factors such as gender, marital status, class, age and ethnicity remain important determinants in people's lives. We have shown that the absence of key social and material resources may override negative perceptions of risk. In our view it is this question of agency and structure that needs more careful delineation in examining perceptions and management of risk in everyday settings. Strong claims about the degree of importance or centrality of risk in late modern life need to be tempered by empirical investigation of how far this is experienced and what impact social contexts have on it. Under these conditions, a more grounded and critical view of risk in everyday life may emerge.

Notes

1. GP records for 28 of the long-term users indicated that they had received a benzodiazepine prescription in seven of the last ten years.
2. It may be that the racist attitudes and practices of some doctors and ancillary staff (Bryan et al. 1985) also help to explain the different patterns of tranquillizer use among black and white women. However, none of the black women in this study said that racism had reduced their willingness to seek medical advice and drug therapy for their personal problems.
3. As Conrad & Schneider (1980) have pointed out medicalization also occurs at a conceptual level, when a medical vocabulary is used to define a problem; and at an institutional level when medical professionals legitimate a programme or problem in which an organization specializes.

References

Ashton, G. & J. Golding 1989. Tranquillisers: prevalence, predictors and possible consequences: data from a large United Kingdom survey. *British Journal of Addiction* **84**, 541–6.

Beck, U. 1992a. *Risk society. Towards a new modernity*. London: Sage.

Beck, U. 1992b. From industrial society to the risk society: questions of survival, social structure and ecological enlightenment. *Theory, Culture and Society* **9**, 97–123.

Bellaby, P. 1990. To risk or not to risk? Uses and limitations of Mary Douglas on risk acceptability for understanding health and safety at work and road accidents. *Sociological Review* **38**, 465–83.

British Broadcasting Corporation (BBC) 1991. The Halcion nightmare. *Panorama*, 14 October.

Brown, P. 1992. Popular epidemiology and toxic waste contamination. *Journal of Health and Social Behaviour* **33**, 267–81.

Bryan, B., S. Dadzie, S. Scafe 1985. *The heart of the race. Black women's lives in Britain*. London: Virago.

Bury, M. & J. Gabe 1990. Hooked? Media responses to tranquillizer dependence. In *New directions in the sociology of health*, P. Abbott & G. Payne (eds), 87–103. London: Falmer.

Calnan, M. & S. Williams 1992. Images of scientific medicine. *Sociology of Health and Illness* **14**, 233–54.

Clinthorne, J. K., I. H. Cisin, M. B. Balter, G. D. Mellinger, E. H. Uhlenhuth 1986. Changes in popular attitudes and beliefs about tranquillizers. *Archives of General Psychiatry* **43**, 527–32.

Cohen, S. 1983. Current attitudes about the benzodiazepines: trial by media. *Journal of Psychoactive Drugs* **15**, 109–13.

Columbia Broadcasting System (CBS) 1991. *60 minutes*, 15 December.

Conrad, P. 1994. Wellness as virtue: morality and the pursuit of health. *Culture, Medicine and Psychiatry* **18**, 385–401.

Conrad, P. & J. W. Schneider 1980. Looking at levels of medicalization: a comment on Strong's critique of the thesis of medical imperialism. *Social Science and Medicine* **14A**, 75–9.

Cooperstock, R. & H. L. Lennard 1979. Some social meanings of tranquilliser use. *Sociology of Health and Illness* **1**, 331–47.

Crawford, R. 1984. A cultural account of "health": control, release and the social body. In *Issues in the political economy of health*, J. B. McKinlay (ed.), 60–103. London: Tavistock.

Curran, V. & S. Golombok 1985. *Bottling it up*. London: Faber & Faber.

Daily Mirror 1982. The dangers of the happiness pill. 11 March.

The Daily Telegraph 1991. Deadlines set for addiction case claims. 5 July.

Davison, C., G. Davey-Smith, S. Frankel 1991. Lay epidemiology and the prevention paradox: the implications of coronary candidacy for health education. *Sociology of Health and Illness* **13**, 1–19.

Department of Health (DoH) (1995) Statistics Division, personal communication.

Douglas, M. 1985. *Risk acceptability according to the social sciences*. London: Routledge.

Elston, M. A. 1994. The anti-vivisectionist movement and the science of medicine. In *Challenging medicine*, J. Gabe, D. Kelleher, G. Williams (eds), 160–80. London: Routledge.

Ettorre, E. 1985. Psychotropics, passivity and the pharmaceutical industry. In *Big deal: the politics of the illicit drugs business*, A. Henman, R. Lewis, T. Maylon (eds). London: Pluto.

Ettorre, E. 1992. *Women and substance use*. Basingstoke: Macmillan.

REFERENCES

Foner, N. 1978. *Jamaica farewell: Jamaican migrants to London*. Berkeley: University of California Press.

Gabe, J. & M. Bury 1988. Tranquillisers as a social problem. *Sociological Review* **36**, 320–52.

Gabe, J. & M. Bury 1991. Tranquillisers and the crisis of health care. *Social Science and Medicine* **32**, 449–54.

Gabe, J. & M. Bury 1994. Halcion nights: a sociological account of a medical controversy. Unpublished paper.

Gabe, J., U. Gustaffson, M. Bury 1991. Mediating illness: newspaper coverage of tranquilliser dependence. *Sociology of Health and Illness* **13**, 332–53.

Gabe, J. & S. Lipshitz-Phillips 1982. Evil necessity? The meaning of benzodiazepine use for women patients from one general practice. *Sociology of Health and Illness* **4**, 201–9.

Gabe, J. & S. Lipshitz-Phillips 1984. Tranquillisers as social control? *Sociological Review* **32**, 524–46.

Gabe, J. & N. Thorogood 1986. Prescribed drugs and the management of everyday life: the experience of black and white working class women. *Sociological Review* **34**, 737–72.

Giddens, A. 1991. *Modernity and self-identity*. Cambridge: Polity.

Giddens, A. 1994. *Beyond left and right*. Cambridge: Polity.

Gordon, B. 1979. *I'm dancing as fast as I can*. New York: Harper & Row.

Guardian 1994. Sad story of the happy pills. 5 April.

Hall, C. 1994. BBC faces £1.5m bill after libel case. *Independent*, 28 May.

Hall, S. 1983. The great moving right show. In *The politics of Thatcherism*, S. Hall & M. Jacques (eds), 19–39. London: Lawrence & Wishart.

Handwerker, L. 1994. Medical risk: implicating poor pregnant women. *Social Science and Medicine* **38**, 665–75.

Helman, C. 1981. "Tonic", "fuel" and "food": social and symbolic aspects of the long-term use of psychotropic drugs. *Social Science and Medicine* **15B**, 521–33.

Holland, J., C. Ramazanoglu, S. Sharpe, R. Thomson 1992. Pleasure, pressure and power: some contradictions of gendered sexuality. *Sociological Review* **40**, 645–73.

Hughes, R. & R. Brewin 1979. *The tranquillizing of America: Pill popping and the American way of life*. New York: Harper & Row.

Independent 1991. Judge gives claim deadline for tranquilliser addiction. 5 July.

King, M., J. Gabe, P. Williams, E. K. Rodrigo 1990. Long term use of benzodiazepines: the views of patients. *British Journal of General Practice* **40**, 194–6.

Koumjian, K. 1981. The use of Valium as a form of social control. *Social Science and Medicine* **15E**, 245–9.

Kramer, P. D. 1993. *Listening to Prozac*. New York: Viking.

Lacey, R. & S. Woodward 1985. *That's Life survey on tranquillisers*. London: BBC Publications.

Linn, L. S. & M. S. Davis 1971. The use of psychotherapeutic drugs by middle-aged women. *Journal of Health and Social Behaviour* **12**, 331–40.

McKeganey, N. & M. Barnard 1992. *AIDS, drugs and sexual risk. Lives in the balance*. Buckingham: Open University Press.

Manheimer, D. I., S. T. Davidson, M. B. Balter, G. D. Mellinger, I. H. Cisin, H. J. Parry 1973. Popular attitudes and beliefs about tranquillizers. *American Journal of Psychiatry* **130**, 1246–53.

Melville, J. 1984. *The tranquillizer trap and how to get out of it.* Glasgow: Fontana.

Montagne, M. 1991. The culture of long-term tranquilliser users. In *Understanding tranquilliser use*, J. Gabe (ed.), 48–68. London: Routledge.

Morley, D. 1992. *Television, audiences and cultural studies.* London: Routledge.

Murray, J. 1981. Long-term psychotropic drug-taking and the process of withdrawal. *Psychological Medicine* **11**, 853–8.

Nelkin, D. 1989. Communicating technological risk: the social construction of risk perception. *Annual Review of Public Health* **10**, 95–113.

Nelkin, D. 1991. Aids and the news media. *The Milbank Quarterly* **69**, 293–307.

Observer 1980a. The dangers of tranquillity. 24 February.

Observer 1980b. Prescription risk. 2 March.

Office of Health Economics (OHE) 1994. *Health information and the consumer. (OHE Briefing No 30).* London: Office of Health Economics.

Parsons, E. & P. Atkinson 1992. Lay constructions of genetic risk. *Sociology of Health and Illness* **14**, 437–55.

Pearson, D. 1981. *Race, class and political activism: a study of West Indians in Britain.* Farnborough: Gower.

Public Citizen Health Research Group 1982. *Stopping Valium.* New York: Pantheon.

Saks, M. 1994. The alternatives to medicine. In *Challenging medicine*, J. Gabe, D. Kelleher, G. Williams (eds), 84–103. London: Routledge.

Short, J. 1984. The social fabric at risk: towards the social transformation of risk analysis. *American Sociological Review* **49**, 711–25.

Silverstone, R. 1994. *Television and everyday life.* London: Routledge.

Standard 1981. Why the happy pills have had their day. 16 October.

Standing, G. 1981. *Unemployment and female labour: a study of labour supply in Kingston Jamaica.* London: Macmillan.

Stone, K. 1983. Motherhood and waged work: West Indian, Asian and white women compared. In *One way ticket: migration and female labour*, A. Phizacklea (ed.), 33–52. London: Routledge & Kegan Paul.

Time 1960. Tranquil but alert. 7 March, 47.

Vogue 1975. Danger ahead! Valium – The pill you love can turn on you. February, 152–3.

Williams, G. & J. Popay 1994. Lay knowledge and the privilege of experience. In *Challenging medicine*, J. Gabe, D. Kelleher, G. Williams (eds), 118–39. London: Routledge.

Young, A. 1976. Some implications of medical beliefs and practices for social anthropology. *American Anthropologist* **78**, 5–24.

Chapter 5

Perceptions and use of anti-hypertensive drugs among cultural groups

Myfanwy Morgan

Introduction

The most common form of treatment in western medicine is the prescribing of pharmaceutical drugs designed to act on specific physiological processes. Seven out of ten general practice consultations in the NHS now end with a prescription being given, and large numbers of people with chronic conditions, such as arthritis, epilepsy and asthma, take medication on a long-term basis (Chew 1992). Thus for many people an important aspect of their illness experience involves managing their treatment. In addition, people are increasingly prescribed drugs for conditions that although not a disease in themselves are identified as a risk factor. A prime example is the treatment of essential hypertension (generally referred to as high blood pressure), with drug therapy being used to control blood pressure levels as a means of reducing risks of coronary heart disease and stroke. This reliance on "medicine" or pills – for curing and even preventing illness, can be viewed as a culturally rooted way of responding to problems of ill health, whose place has been taken in other societies and historical periods by natural remedies, magical potions or spirit invocation. Indeed the use of the term "medicines" to refer to pharmaceutical drugs, emphasizes their key position and status in western medicine.

Pharmaceutical drugs not only serve an instrumental function within modern biomedicine but are also invested with a symbolic significance within the lay culture. As Montagne (1988) observes, the original Greek term for drug, "pharmakon" has three meanings, remedy, poison and magical charm, which still appear to be present in everyday metaphors and images of drugs. The notion of the magical ability of drugs is to some extent retained and reflected in the discovery of "magic bullets" or the "miracle drugs" of the 1930s and 1940s, the antibiotics, which provided rapid and effective cures for conditions that were previously associated with high levels of morbidity. Furthermore even though modern medicine is deemed rational and scientific, a certain magic and mysticism often envelops the drugs that health professionals use, in that they are the visible sign of the physician's power to heal and may express the healer's knowledge and concern. Thus the prescribing of drugs often serves a symbolic function in the consultation, communicating the physician's concern for the patient's problem. People's faith in the power of drugs may also in itself be beneficial. This is acknowledged in terms of the placebo effect, which literally means "I will please" and refers to the finding that as much as one-third of the effects of prescribed medication can be attributed to its meanings for patients rather than to its chemical substances (Beecher 1955). Thus the power of drugs partly derives from the perception of them as a symbol of healing, and is often associated with a more general faith in medicine and doctors.

In contrast to these positive images of drugs as "cure", "remedy" and "magic" are the images of drugs as "death", "disease", "plague", and "scourge" (Montagne 1988). Even when used in a therapeutic context, drugs may cause rather than cure disease by producing adverse reactions with an estimated 240,000 hospitalizations in Britain per year believed to result wholly or partly from drugs (Davies 1981). By the end of the 1980s it was also estimated that about half a million people in Britain were more or less addicted to benzodiazepines (Medawar 1992). Concern about harmful side-effects of drugs and inappropriate prescribing are thus common themes in the medical literature. More broadly, the high level of prescribing of licit psychotropic drugs relates to what for Illich (1976) is a central aspect of the medicalization of life, in terms of the society's over-dependence on drugs to induce sleep, and to treat grief, depression and other "problems of living". Such reliance is viewed as a modern scourge that produces both adverse clinical effects (drug-induced illness) and the expropriation of individual's and communities' coping abilities, self-reliance and autonomy.

Prevailing social images and meanings of pharmaceutical drugs are conveyed by the media who present newsworthy stories of new "miracle" drugs, and drug "disasters", such as the Thalidomide tragedy in the 1960s, the effects of Opren among elderly people in the 1980s, and scares about the contraceptive pill. A continuing theme is also provided by medical stories of dependence on licit and illicit psychotropic drugs that depict the devastating nature of tranquillizers as all powerful and controlling their users. In this way the media exert a powerful influence not only in communicating information but also in shaping images and meanings of drugs in the lay culture, with the messages conveyed being influenced by journalists' desire to dramatize, simplify and personalize their stories in the context of the prevailing cultural frameworks (see Gabe et al. 1991 and Ch. 4).

The dual image of drugs in the lay culture in terms of both their beneficial and harmful effects is reflected in patients' ideas and assessments of prescribed medications. Thus while valuing the benefits of prescribed drugs in controlling symptoms and reducing risks of asthma attacks, epileptic fits or other adverse effects, patients also frequently express concerns about possible harmful effects of the drugs and fears of becoming "addicted" to or dependent on the drugs (Conrad 1985, Donovan & Blake 1992). There is thus evidence of a lack of complete faith and endorsement of medicine by the lay or patient population. More generally, at any one time there are likely to be variations in what Cornwell (1984) refers to as "medicalization from below", or the degree of acceptance of modern scientific medicine among different social groups. As noted in earlier chapters, there is evidence of differences in acceptance of the authority of medicine and its remedies among different groups in the population, with younger and middle-class people tending to be more sceptical about drugs and medical technology than older people and those from a working-class background, which may reflect a greater willingness among younger age groups and higher social classes to be critical of the authority of medicine and scientific knowledge. However, perhaps of greater significance is the presence of ethnic minorities who are to some extent outside the dominant culture and its system of meanings. Their self-identity or sense of "peoplehood" is associated with a common homeland or land of origin, and the maintenance of aspects of a distinctive culture, in terms of their social institutions (religion, family structures and marriage), social norms, manners, attitudes, ways of thinking and social behaviours (diet, dress, health practices). Although ethnic minorities are often viewed as a single category or collective in terms of their common experiences of migration and differences from the wider society, they nevertheless form distinct groups with their own history, identity, circumstances and culture, as well as in the extent of their integration and adoption of the beliefs and practices of the wider society.

This chapter examines the significance of ethnicity for "white" and Afro-Caribbean patients' beliefs and responses to a specific treatment modality, namely the use of anti-hypertensive drugs. These drugs are prescribed to lower blood pressures that are above a threshold regarded as comprising a significantly increased risk of cardiovascular events. Blood pressures at the higher end of the distribution thus constitute a graded risk factor rather than a disease and have been "medicalized" on the basis that elevations in blood pressure are associated with increased risks of heart disease and stroke. However, thresholds for treatment have varied in response to prevailing medical views of the benefits of risk reduction compared with the costs to patients of taking drugs regularly for an asymptomatic condition (Kwachi & Wilson 1990). Lowering blood pressure through drug treatment, weight control, dietary changes and other lifestyle measures now forms a major preventive strategy, given that heart disease and stroke rank first and third as major causes of death and accounted for 26 per cent and 12 per cent respectively of deaths in England, in 1991 (Secretary of State 1993). Indeed the large number of people who can be regarded as at significantly increased risk of cardiovascular disease has meant that high blood pressure now forms the most common reason for initiating life-long drug therapy in modern industrial societies. There is concern as to the high proportion of patients dropping out of treatment altogether, and of the irregular use of drugs among many remaining in treatment (Hart 1987). However, although high blood pressure has been the subject of a large number of medically oriented studies investigating the "problem" of patients' "non-compliance" with drug treatment, little is known about how patients themselves perceive anti-hypertensive drug treatment, nor of the possible variations among ethnic groups.

One marker of the cultural integration of ethnic minorities in the health field and the extent of their medicalization is whether they continue to use herbal and other traditional remedies as well as western drug treatments, and thus participate in a dual system of health care. There is evidence that poorer sections of the Asian community in the UK continue to use proprietary and herbal remedies and Asian healers are known to practice in some cities, whereas more educated middle-class sections of the Asian community rely entirely on western medicines (Bhopal 1986, Donovan 1986). Similarly, many of the older generation of Afro-Caribbean people in the UK continue to use herbal remedies, although the younger generation appears to be rejecting this tradition (Donovan 1986, Thorogood 1990). Herbal remedies are thus of significance for some sections of the ethnic minority population and can be conceptualized as an additional "resource", that along with other material and socio-cultural resources are differentially available and utilized in managing people's everyday lives and problems of illness (Gabe & Thorogood 1986). However, herbal remedies may not only complement or serve as an alternative to prescribed drugs but may also be associated with a continuation of traditional belief systems and meanings that shape how ethnic minority groups perceive western drug treatments. Thus a process of what Herskovits (1948) describes as "cultural re-interpretation" may occur in which traditional meanings are ascribed to new elements, with modern treatments of western medicine being placed within a traditional explanatory framework and system of healing, rather than accompanied by "medicalization" and acceptance of the cultural meanings prevalent in western society and western medicine. However, as Bledsoe & Gaubard (1985) observe, because of our own familiarity with these objects, we may often fail to perceive that this shift in meanings has taken place.

Even within our own society there is a tendency to assume uncritically a single set of meanings, based on the premise that the meanings and assumptions of the medical profession are necessarily shared by patients. This is reflected particularly strongly in relation to investigations of patients' medication use that have traditionally reflected a medical ideology that requires patient "compliance", and is justified in terms of what are assumed to be the beneficial effects to patients of the prescribed drugs. The only medically acceptable reason for patients' non-compliance is the experience of side-effects, which may require a simple change in the drugs or dose prescribed. Otherwise, patients' non-compliance is viewed as "default" and explained in terms of patients' forgetting, or their lack of understanding or knowledge about their drug regime, drug actions, or medical condition (Becker 1985, Roth 1987). In contrast to this approach a small number of studies adopting an interpretive perspective have acknowledged the differing realities of doctors and patients and examined patients' own beliefs and practices in relation to long-term medication use (Conrad 1985, Hunt et al. 1989, Donovan & Blake 1992). These studies depict patients as thoughtful decision-makers whose medication use is influenced by the culturally shaped meanings attributed to the prescribed drugs and to their medical condition, as well as by patients' personal meanings based on their own experiences, priorities and evaluations in the context of their everyday life and activities. Drugs prescribed by the doctor are thus perceived, evaluated and responded to within the patient's own "illness" framework, rather than a medical "disease" framework (Eisenberg 1977). However, despite this recognition of the importance of patients' meanings and of the ways in which such meanings are shaped by the broader lay culture and patients' own circumstances and resources, little attention has been paid to the meanings of prescribed drugs held by ethnic groups in the UK. Thus the question arises as to whether the beliefs and treatment practices of ethnic minorities correspond with those of the wider patient population and thus form one aspect of what Kleinman (1980) refers to as a shared "explanatory model" or understanding of disease, illness and treatment, or whether drug treatments are "re-interpreted" and responded to within traditional cultural frameworks.

Afro-Caribbean and white hypertensive patients

People from the Caribbean comprise the second biggest ethnic group in the UK, accounting for 500,000 people or 0.9 per cent of the population

(Teague 1993). Small numbers of people from the Caribbean have lived in Britain since the early years of this century, with settlements occurring around the ports of Liverpool and Cardiff associated with colonial trade. However, the major migration occurred in the period in the 1950s to early 1960s in response to the job opportunities during the period of reconstruction and labour shortage in the UK. Most of these early migrants are thus now aged between 50 and 65 years, and experience a relatively high prevalence of hypertension and stroke as do their counterparts in the Caribbean (Beevers & Beevers 1993). Large numbers are therefore being treated with anti-hypertensive drugs to control their blood pressure.

The present research formed part of a larger study of patients' and doctors' meanings and management of high blood pressure, and was based on 15 general practices in the London borough of Lambeth that has the highest concentration of Afro-Caribbean people (12.6 per cent) of any district in the UK. The criteria employed in recruiting "white" and Afro-Caribbean hypertensive patients were that they were aged at least 35 years, in a manual occupation group (to "match" for similar socio-economic position), treated for hypertension for at least one year (to allow stable patterns to have developed), and not treated for any other chronic condition. Major reasons for exclusion were the frequent association of diabetes and high blood pressure among Afro-Caribbean patients, and the aim of recruiting similar numbers of white and Afro-Caribbean patients from each study practice. The target of 60 patient interviews (30 "white" and 30 Afro-Caribbean), equally divided between men and women was achieved from an initial group of 72 patient names (83 per cent), with no contact being made with nine people. The 60 respondents were all interviewed in their own homes using a semi-structured approach. All interviews were tape-recorded and later transcribed. Themes and explanations were then identified through content analysis of the transcripts.

The 30 "white" respondents were all born in England apart from three people who had come from southern Ireland over 10 years ago. The Afro-Caribbean respondents were all born in the Caribbean, all except two in Jamaica. They had come to Britain as young adults during the period from the 1950s to early 1960s in response to the job opportunities and settled in south London, reflecting the general pattern of Afro-Caribbean migration to the UK. Their early experience in the Caribbean was of a culture that was strongly influenced and shaped by the white and predominantly British colonial settlers, and involved a common language, religion, educational and health system, as well as a common affinity with Britain as the "mother" country (Goulbourne 1991). They have now lived in the UK for over 30 years but often continue to eat traditional foods, such as salt fish and yams, and maintain other aspects of their culture in terms of forms of church worship and music, etc., and often regard the Caribbean (or their particular island) as "home". Their social environment and culture thus reflect an amalgam of their Afro-Caribbean traditions and the dominant values and institutions in Britain.

The white and Afro-Caribbean respondents all lived in the same areas of inner London, often in council-rented flats on large estates, and were attending the same general practices. They also shared a similar socio-economic situation. One-quarter of the men in both groups were unemployed and common occupations among the employed were caretaker, railway worker, general labourer and factory worker. Most women worked either full or part-time, often as clerical workers, cleaners, cashiers and shop assistants. They were thus drawn from an economically disadvantaged sector of the population with the only major differences between groups relating to their ethnicity.

The white and Afro-Caribbean respondents had all been prescribed anti-hypertensive drugs for at least one year and almost one-half had been treated for over five years. To some extent they thus form a self-selected group in that they had all formally continued under treatment, whereas large numbers of people are known to drop out of treatment altogether, especially during the first year (Hart 1987). They had also had time to reach a stage of longer-term adjustment to this condition and acquire knowledge of its nature and effects.

The term "high blood pressure" was used throughout the interviews in preference to "hypertension" as although patients are generally familiar with the term hypertension they do not always regard it as the same as high blood pressure (Blumhagen 1980, Morgan & Watkins 1988). In accord with the status of high blood pressure as a risk factor, it was notable that everyone rejected the view of themselves as "ill" , or "sick", and often explained that despite their blood pressure problem they were able to lead a normal life and do things as usual. However, they were aware of and often commented on their rather ambivalent status of being "under the doctor" for blood pressure and prescribed drug treatment but not "sick". For example, a white woman described herself as:

> Delicate – no not delicate – I can't think of the word for it. I wouldn't say I'm an ill person, but I wouldn't like to say I'm healthy. I don't know whether that makes sense really. You feel as though it's always there, but it doesn't affect you (02).

She explained that, "I don't think I've changed anything. I still go to work. I go for walks". However, she also acknowledged that she did not over-exert herself in case it was bad for her blood pressure, and does not now run for a bus.

An Afro-Caribbean man similarly described himself as:

Not ill, but I can't be 100 per cent well as I've got this blood pressure and I'm under the doctor (12).

He then explained that with his blood pressure he had not got much energy to come in from work and do the gardening, and had to take things easy.

These notions of taking things more easily, either because rushing around and getting tired or stressed was bad for your blood pressure or because having blood pressure meant you lacked energy, were common themes. They appeared to form a major part of the impact of high blood pressure on people's everyday life and activities and people's interpretation of this condition. This concern not to rush around and avoid stress as a means of blood pressure control corresponds with patients' perceptions of stress as a major cause of high blood pressure as well as leading to temporary elevations in blood pressure (Blumhagen 1980, Morgan & Watkins 1988).

The respondents were all aware that having high blood pressure meant that they were at increased risk of death, and all but three identified themselves as at increased risk of a heart attack or stroke. However, only one-third mentioned both conditions. The white respondents were most likely to identify themselves as at risk of heart problems, with 22 mentioning this and 16 mentioning a stroke, whereas 18 Afro-Caribbean respondents mentioned heart problems and 24 a stroke. This differing emphasis reflects the relative importance of these conditions in the two communities, with death rates for stroke being much higher among Afro-Caribbeans and rates of coronary heart disease relatively low compared with the general population of England and Wales (Balarajan 1991). However, although people were aware of these risks, when asked if there was any condition they thought they might get only 16 of the 60 respondents mentioned any condition and just eight people identified a stroke or heart problem. These eight people all had close relatives who had died of a stroke. The majority therefore did not feel personally vulnerable to a heart attack or stroke, with this often being influenced by their faith in the tablets to control their blood pressure or the knowledge that it was under control. It was also notable that the Afro-Caribbean respondents were aware that high blood pressure was common among their people and appeared to derive some reassurance from the prevalence or "normality" of this condition.

Perceptions and use of drug treatment

One-third of the respondents in each ethnic group said that their drugs had been changed in the past because of problems of headache, nausea dizziness and other recognized side-effects. Many people are also likely to have dropped out of treatment for this reason. The experience of drug side-effects was not currently said to be a problem. However, there may have been some under-reporting of this, especially in terms of the recognized effects of beta blockers in causing impotence that was only acknowledged by two men. A number of other people also described symptoms that they thought might be related to the drugs such as tiredness, dizziness and headaches, but were unsure whether they were caused by the drugs or by their blood pressure, or if they were merely part of growing old and thus "normal" in these terms. As these respondents explained:

I get headaches quite a lot but I'm not saying whether that's the blood pressure or not doing that. I always get tired a bit, but I don't know if that's to do with the tablets or not (39).

I couldn't really tell you. I wouldn't know for sure. But I do get giddy spells but I don't know what's causing it. I don't think I get any problems from the tablets (36).

Interpretation of current symptoms and evaluation of the drugs was thus problematic for patients in view of the difficulties in assigning cause and effect.

In terms of current medication use, only 12 of the 30 Afro-Caribbean patients said they took the drugs regularly as prescribed, two often forgot and 16 took the drugs irregularly or took a reduced dose. In contrast, only two of the 30 white patients acknowledged that they did not take the drugs regularly and a further two patients had recently been taken off the drugs by their general practitioners, whereas 26 respondents said they took the drugs regularly. This high level of regular medication use reported by the white respondents corresponds with the findings of a recent study by Gilbert et al. (1990) based on hypertensive patients attending community clinics in Australia, and may partly reflect the effects of selective processes, as many patients are likely to have dropped out of treatment with those remaining forming a self-selected group. It is also recognized that their reported medication use may not have corresponded with their actual everyday medication practices, as patients may overestimate their medication use in situations where they believe that acknowledging "non-compliance" would be regarded unfavourably (Becker 1985). Questions regarding drug use were therefore prefaced in the study by acknowledging that patients often do not take drugs as prescribed by the doctor, to convey the acceptability of reporting such behaviour rather than the need to present a "public" account, or behaviour that accords with medical expectations. The patients who reported taking the medication regularly as prescribed frequently offered to show the interviewer their tablets and conveyed their genuineness by the nature and definiteness of their responses. For example, they described themselves in terms such as "a model patient", "rarely missing if ever" and as taking the tablets "religiously everyday". They also recounted their strategies and routines for remembering, including taking the tablets at set times, being helped to remember by their spouse, and keeping a reserve supply at a convenient place such as at work. Some people did however acknowledge that they might occasionally forget if routines were disrupted, particularly at weekends and holidays. As might be expected, problems of remembering were greatest for people who were required to take tablets two or three times a day rather than just once.

Patients who described themselves as taking the medications as prescribed can be classified as displaying "stable" adherence or "problematic" adherence in terms of the extent to which they were reconciled to taking the drugs as prescribed. Altogether 16 of the 26 white respondents who took the medication as prescribed and eight of the 12 Afro-Caribbean respondents may be characterized as displaying "stable" adherence. This consisted of people who were taking the medication as prescribed, and who did not express any major worries or concerns about taking the tablets or possibly having to remain on them all their life. They would have preferred not to take the tablets and were aware that taking the tablets signified that they were not perfectly healthy, but their general view was that taking blood pressure tablets was a small price to pay for reducing their risks of stroke or heart disease and they appeared to have reconciled themselves to this. As one man who had been treated for blood pressure for three years explained:

> It doesn't bother me whether I have to take them all my life or not. If it's going to keep me alive then I've got to take them. That's how I look at it (44).

Similarly a woman currently took the view that:

> To pop a little pink pill in my mouth, there's a lot worse things that you have to cope with everyday. No it doesn't bother me at all (16).

However, she acknowledged that three years ago when she first started treatment and ran out of tablets she stopped taking them for a while. As a result, when she next went to be checked by the general practitioner her blood pressure was found to be elevated and she was told off by the doctor. The effect of this was that she changed her medication practices so that, "Now I always take them everyday. It's a regular routine I've got, it's a habit like anything else."

This move from being an irregular to a regular user was also described by other respondents. The main reason for their change in medication practice was that their blood pressure had gone up, and they were warned by the doctor and told severely about the need to take the tablets regularly. This illustrates the way in which patterns of medication use and views about drugs may evolve and change over time in response to new information of circumstances, rather than forming the static category that often characterizes the medical literature.

In contrast to the "stable" adherents both the "problematic" adherents (10 white and four Afro-Caribbean respondents) and those not taking the drugs as prescribed (two white and 18 Afro-Caribbean respondents) appeared less reconciled to taking the drugs and mentioned concerns about current or anticipated adverse effects. This took a number of forms. Two men mentioned problems of the drugs causing impotence, although this concern may in reality have been more widespread. Another problem mentioned by four Afro-Caribbean men was that "drugs and alcohol don't mix". They thought that if they took both they might go into a coma or die, and would therefore not take the drugs if they were planning to go to a party and drink spirits (mainly rum) over the weekend:

> I am a man that goes out to parties sometimes and has a nice drink. When you are taking drugs you have to limit your drinks. If I know that I'm going out on a Saturday night or Friday or Sunday I won't take the tablets as you do not want to mix the drugs with the alcohol.

> Interviewer: Why is that?

> It is not something you should do, you can die if you mix them (55).

A major concern about the drugs that was mentioned by both men and women in both ethnic groups related to worries about anticipated future "side-effects". As two white respondents explained:

> I have thought about side-effects. If you keep on with these tablets, what is it going to do eventually? That's what bothers me (5).

> It bothers me taking the tablets long-term because I do not know what the long-term effects of the tablets will be. I do not think anybody does (40).

Similar observations were made by Afro-Caribbean respondents:

> I used to say to my friend at work that these tablets are going to affect my insides. She said don't be silly . . . Taking so much of them each day and for so long, they might do something to me (32).

> I see too many people on tablets having side-effects, so I try and get away from tablets, not to take them. I must be really bad to take the tablets because I don't like tablets (30).

This concern about "side-effects" refers to what can be regarded as adverse reactions, or side-effects of an unexpected and sometimes serious nature. Fallsberg (1991) notes that in Sweden where there is only a single word for side-effects a distinction is made in professional circles between Type A and Type B side-effects. Type A are the predictable, normal pharmacological effects of a drug given in a therapeutic dose and consist of well-known reactions that are often due to the inadequate selectivity of preparations, whereas Type B refers to unexpected serious side-effects that are difficult to predict and which appear to form the basis of these respondents' concerns.

The other main reason for people's dislike of the drugs was a fear of being "addicted" to or dependent on the drugs and unable to do without them. This characterized both ethnic groups but appeared to be of particular concern to the Afro-Caribbean respondents. As one Afro-Caribbean respondent explained when asked about taking the tablets:

> Sometimes I remember and sometimes I do not because I don't want to build my hopes on tablets. I don't want to become an addict (29).

Similarly a white respondent when asked whether it bothered him having to take the tablets explained:

> Well it does really. It sounds like you're being hooked onto a blood pressure tablet . . . It bothers me taking tablets all the time but you need this one tablet to keep your blood pressure down (19).

These concerns about possible anticipated harmful effects of drugs and a dislike of feeling dependent on drugs reflect general aspects of the beliefs and meaning of drugs within the lay culture and are commonly expressed by patients. Whether such concerns lead to people stopping treatment altogether, reducing the dosage or irregular drug use, will be influenced by the strength of these concerns, and patients' assessment of the seriousness of their condition and the benefits of taking the drugs. The main benefit for people with high blood pressure is to reduce their risk of a heart attack or stroke and their worries about this. Perception of these benefits is likely to have been the reason why some respondents who expressed concerns about having to take the drugs nevertheless said they did take them regularly as prescribed. They thus displayed "problematic" adherence, in that although taking the tablets regularly, they were not reconciled to long-term use of anti-hypertensive drugs and still worried about possible harmful effects in the future or expressed a dislike of feeling "addicted" to the drugs. Rather than engage in "problematic" adherence, the main response to such concerns among most Afro-Caribbean patients, was to take the drugs irregularly. Two respondents took a reduced dose and 14 regularly "left off" the drugs. "Leaving off" the drugs took two forms. Some people "left off" the drugs for a few days each week on a regular basis, with the aim of reducing their total intake of drugs, and thus the risks of harmful "side-effects" or becoming "addicted" to the drugs. For example, respondent 29, quoted earlier, took the drugs only on alternate days to avoid becoming dependent on them. Other people "left off" the drugs for several weeks or months at a time if they were feeling all right:

I prefer to let nature take its course as far as my body is concerned. I'm not one to introduce anything to it if I'm feeling all right. If I'm feeling ill I will take any medication that will make me better or even cure me, but if I feel better I don't see why I should take it, because I don't want to be addicted to nothing other than food and water (50).

This respondent also explained that if told his blood pressure was high he would take the drugs, but "Only if I was feeling bad all the time. If I was feeling fine for a day or two then maybe I would miss a day or two. If that's cheating on myself then that's it."

Another respondent who "left off" the drugs for long periods also commented:

Please don't tell him (Dr) this, but I'm a person that if I find it's stable and I'm not getting any funny feelings then I don't take them. If I feel peaky again, then I go back on them.

Interviewer: Why don't you take them?

You know that people get hooked on all these drugs and then you can't do without them . . . I always thought to myself that I really don't want to live a life where I have to swallow down tablets. That's why when I'm not feeling too bad I don't take them to see that my body can function without a heap of tablets going down (58).

Although many Afro-Caribbean patients "left off" the drugs they were aware that they were expected to take the medication regularly. They were also concerned about their blood pressure and visited their doctor to have it checked. The high level of non-adherence among Afro-Caribbean patients thus did not appear to reflect conventional medical explanations of "non-compliance". However, it was associated with uncontrolled and fluctuating blood pressures. Although general practitioners had often changed their tablets to achieve better blood pressure control, the most recent reading recorded in patients' case notes indicated that 16 Afro-Caribbean patients and ten white patients had uncontrolled pressures of 100 mm Hg diastolic and over and included five Afro-Caribbean patients with extremely high blood pressure of 110 mm Hg diastolic or above. This latter group were all taking the drugs irregularly and at this blood pressure level experienced a significantly increased risk of cardiovascular disease. It thus appeared that Afro-Caribbean patients' medication practices were of significance for their blood pressure control, while their irregular drug use and particular concerns about the prescribed medications raise questions regarding the influence of traditional remedies and explanatory frameworks for their responses to the prescribed drugs.

Significance of traditional remedies

Herbal remedies continued to be taken by 17 of the 30 Afro-Caribbean respondents, including most of the people who "left off" the drugs. Most people took herbal remedies as a general tonic or to "cleanse the system", whereas some were taking them specifically for their blood pressure. Such distinctions cannot however be clearly drawn, as the same herbal remedies are often used for many purposes. For example, the herbal remedy cerasee was most frequently mentioned by the respondents, and generally described as good for reducing blood pressure. However, cerasee was also taken for a number of other conditions including stomach aches, as a wash-out to cleanse the system, and as a general tonic to promote good health. A bottled herbal drink, Constitution Bitters, which is a blend of seven herbs, was also being taken by some respondents, and is described on the label as suitable for high blood pressure, biliousness, loss of appetite and general debility. This use of the same remedy for what in western medicine form discrete diseases with their specific remedies, reflects the association of herbal remedies with humoral theories that regard most illnesses as caused by "cold", "gas or wind", "heat", "bile", "blood imbalances" or "germs". These are each associated with particular herbal remedies that are taken to treat a variety of symptoms (Mitchell 1983).

Herbal remedies were mainly purchased in dried form from the local market that caters for the Afro-Caribbean community in south London, although people said that they also asked relations and friends to bring back some of the fresh herbs from Jamaica where they pick the leaves of various plants and herbs growing wild. Both men and women continued to take herbal remedies, but there was some evidence that the women used a wider variety of folk treatments. Particular remedies mentioned by women included boiling grapefruit skins with garlic and drinking the water, which was regarded as helpful for keeping blood pressure down, and for diabetes and reducing weight. Boiling a piece of sinkelweiss in water was also regarded as very effective in reducing blood pressure. However, the use of this and other traditional remedies was often limited by their lack of availability in the UK, as this respondent explains:

> There are lots of things you get in the West Indies that you can't get over here. You can go up to the mountains and pick herbs, charney root and bloodweiss. You boil them altogether with watergrass.
>
> Interviewer: Is that what you would use for your blood pressure if you were still living in the West Indies?
>
> Yes, all those things brings your pressure right down (21).

Herbal remedies for many people thus formed an additional resource that they took either as well as, or instead of, the prescribed drugs. However, the influence of herbal remedies also appeared to extend more broadly in terms of providing an interpretive framework within which modern medicine was viewed. Thus concerns about the possible harmful effects of prescribed drugs appeared to be exacerbated by their familiarity with herbal remedies, which were regarded as having the advantages of being "natural" substances and therefore less powerful and potentially harmful compared with the prescribed drugs. The practice of "leaving off" the drugs for a few days each week was thus intended to reduce the amount of drugs taken, with the aim of reducing the harmful effects of these powerful substances. Mitchell (1983) notes that within herbal traditions the effectiveness of remedies also tends to be assessed in relation to their effects on symptoms, and are thus not regarded as necessary once the symptom has been alleviated. This concept was also evident in respondents' accounts (e.g. case Nos. 50 and 58), with a major reason for "leaving off" the drugs for long periods being the absence of symptoms and feeling all right, as well as a dislike of feeling dependent on drugs.

One important trigger causing people to start taking the drugs again or to take them more regularly, was being told by their general practitioner that their blood pressure had gone up or was "high". The other was their own feeling that their blood pressure was up. Although high blood pressure is regarded as an asymptomatic condition it has been shown that large numbers of patients feel they can tell when their blood pressure is high (Meyer et al. 1985). In the present study this perception was associated with the experience of symptoms such as pains or "sensations" in their head or neck, feelings of weakness or tiredness, eye problems, dizziness, or feeling hot that were reported by 20 Afro-Caribbean respondents and 15 white respondents. The high prevalence of these symptoms may reflect problems of inadequate blood pressure control, the irregular use of the tablets or side-effects of the tablets, as well as possibly an increased tendency among hypertensive patients to perceive such symptoms and attribute them to blood pressure. The general response by both white and Afro-Caribbean patients was to rest and relax for a time. However the Afro-Caribbean respondents would also start taking the prescribed tablets regularly if these had been "left off" or the dosage reduced. They described this use of the medication as "being taken like a tranquillizer, and not how it's supposed to be", thus demonstrating their own perception of the way in which they were using the drugs in treating symptoms and their awareness of how they were expected to be taken.

Whereas herbal remedies appeared to form an important resource for Afro-Caribbean people who frequently "left off" the prescribed drugs, this form of treatment was dismissed and rejected by the group of Afro-Caribbean respondents who took the blood pressure tablets regularly and were classified as "stable" adherents. For example, one Afro-Caribbean man explained when asked if he thought herbal remedies could help his blood pressure:

> Some people feel it does, but you could be taking something and thinking you're doing yourself good but you're not. It's not the right thing. They made the tablets for these things, so it's best to take the tablets (28).

Similarly, another Afro-Caribbean respondent explained:

The West Indians are great people for herbs but I don't believe in it.

Interviewer: So you have not taken herbal remedies for your blood pressure?

No I don't believe in it. I think if there's going to be an answer to blood pressure, then it's going to come from the lab (11).

These respondents had thus rejected traditional herbal remedies and relied entirely on drug treatments. However, it is not clear why some people had undergone this medicalization and others retained important aspects of traditional beliefs and remedies. This may reflect differences in their experiences in the Caribbean and possibly greater access to a formal health system and western treatments. During the 1950s formal health care in Jamaica was provided by publicly funded hospital services and by general practitioners on a fee for service basis. Access to western health care was thus fairly limited for people living in rural areas who would often have difficulty in reaching the hospital, and for those unable to afford to consult a general practitioner with problems of illness, thus being perceived and responded to by such groups in terms of traditional cultural frameworks and treatments.

Cultural meanings, continuity and change

The notion of the positive and negative effects of drugs was clearly evident in the majority of the accounts of this group of patients on long-term anti-hypertensive drug treatment. Faith in the positive effects of the anti-hypertensive drugs in reducing risks of disease formed the prime reason for patients remaining under treatment, with knowledge of the efficacy of the drugs in controlling their blood pressure also reducing their worries about this condition. Negative perceptions of the drugs mainly related to worries about anticipated harmful effects and concerns about being dependent on or "addicted" to the drugs. These dual meanings and concerns are common in the lay culture and among patient groups in western medical systems. As Fallsberg (1991) observed "Few people are indifferent when faced with the effects of drugs. A yearning for the anticipated effect and fear of side-effects are combined with the air of mystery surrounding the effects of medicines. For people in general, drugs are more than a neutral form of treatment . . . " (p.41). However, there was no evidence that drug treatment for high blood pressure was invested with any special social significance, nor that this condition currently provoked

111

a high level of anxiety among this group of patients who had mainly been under treatment for several years.

An important difference between ethnic groups was that the Afro-Caribbean patients appeared to be less reconciled to taking the tablets compared with their white counterparts, and large numbers of Afro-Caribbean patients did not take the drugs regularly as prescribed. This appeared to be partly associated with the availability of herbal remedies as a resource and their use by some people specifically to control blood pressure. However, of greater significance was their interpretation of the prescribed drugs in terms of their traditional illness–treatment framework or "explanatory model". Important aspects of this included the significance they attached to symptoms in assessing the need for treatment. This accords with the emphasis of traditional humoral theories in which symptoms are equated with disease, rather than being perceived as a manifestation of disease (Mitchell 1983). Thus for people who "left off" the drugs, especially over long periods, their main use of the prescribed drugs appeared to be in responding to symptoms, including knowledge of elevations in their blood pressure, rather than as a preventive measure, despite their awareness of their doctors' recommendations and of the reasons for long-term drug use. Underlying this approach was also their perception of the powerful and thus potentially harmful nature of modern medicines in contrast with traditional remedies, which are regarded as "natural" and therefore as relatively mild. Thus, whereas drugs were viewed favourably for short-term use by Afro-Caribbean patients, they were often reluctant to take drugs on a long-term basis and when they were feeling "all right". This appears to be a common interpretation and response to modern drug remedies among people familiar with traditional herbal treatments that act more slowly. For example, Sussman (1988) found that western drug treatments in Mauritius were acceptable for illnesses requiring rapid relief of symptoms or the killing of germs, whereas for illnesses such as rheumatism, hypertension, palpitations, and diabetes that are either recurrent or chronic and which require long-term medication use, it was believed that drug remedies were too strong to be taken for long periods of time. For such conditions herbal remedies were preferred or might be alternated with biochemical remedies so as to give the body a rest from western medicine. Sachs & Tomson (1992) in their study of drug utilization in Sri Lanka, similarly observed that people had definite ideas about how western medicine works and often used it according to traditional medical theories and practices. Thus although western medicine often exists as an alternative or complementary treatment strategy to traditional remedies, this does not mean that the ideology of western medicine, including its explanations of disease and the meanings of recommended treatment modalities have necessarily been fully accepted. Instead the disease categories of western medicine that themselves form cultural constructs, are reinterpreted and responded to on the basis of these differing meanings.

The maintenance by large numbers of Afro-Caribbean patients of aspects of their traditional cultural beliefs and practices has occurred despite their having lived in the UK and experienced a culture and health system based on western scientific medicine for over 30 years. This cultural continuity is likely to have been reinforced by the geographical concentration of Afro-Caribbean people in particular areas of London, and is associated with the availability of herbal remedies and other products from the Caribbean in local markets. Also of importance is the informal support and advice received from other people with a shared cultural origin and background. Residential proximity thus contributes to the continuation of cultural practices and the maintenance of a sense of self-identity, with similar patterns and the continued use of traditional remedies also characterizing poorer Asian groups in the UK (Bhopal 1986) and some migrant groups in the USA (Harwood 1981).

The group of Afro-Caribbean patients interviewed is distinctive in being drawn from the original migrants who were brought up in the Caribbean, a group that currently comprises 46 per cent of Afro-Caribbeans in the UK (Smaje 1995). Their children were described as rejecting herbal remedies, and presumably were also not familiar with other aspects of traditional explanations of illness. Such intergenerational changes are common, with the children of migrants generally undergoing a process of "medicalization" as one aspect of a more general adoption of the beliefs, practices and lifestyle of the wider culture. The meanings of ethnicity and the composition of groups is therefore fluid, and associated with considerable intra and inter-ethnic variability in health beliefs and practices. In particular it was notable that even this older generation of Afro-Caribbean patients drawn from a manual occupational group was not characterized by a homogeneous set of beliefs, with some people displaying beliefs and practices conforming with the lay culture of western medicine.

Whereas the health beliefs and practices of ethnic minorities are increasingly shaped and influenced by western medicine, there is evidence of an increasing questioning of aspects of modern medicine among the wider lay population. This was represented among the white hypertensive patients interviewed in terms of their concerns regarding the possible adverse effects of long-term drug use and what was characterized as "problematic" adherence. Although the group of white hypertensive patients were not taking alternative remedies for this condition, this may form a response among some patients who drop out of anti-hypertensive drug treatment and especially among people in the higher socio-economic groups. Thus in general there is evidence of an increasing use of alternative therapies such as homeopathy, acupuncture, osteopathy and herbalism, especially among younger and middle-class people (see Sharma 1990 and Ch. 11). These treatments are mainly used to complement biomedicine, with one reason for their use being when biomedical treatments are feared to be too radical or invasive, or drugs are perceived as habit-forming or having undesirable side-effects. There are thus currently movements both to medicalize and de-medicalize in terms of the adoption or rejection of the beliefs and practices of biomedicine among various sections of the lay population, rather than a single uniform trend. This has possible implications for the boundaries of conventional or professionally legitimated medical treatments, especially as demands increase for moving beyond conventional drug treatments to embrace what are currently alternative therapies outside the professional medical sphere. However, changes currently taking place involve not only the "demystification of medicine from below", but also changes in "medicalization from above". For example, recent scientific papers have questioned the need for long-term drug therapy to treat hypertension and present evidence to demonstrate that normal blood pressure once attained may be maintained in the absence of treatment (Fletcher et al. 1988). There is also increasing interest among some medical professionals in the use of yoga, biofeedback and various forms of relaxation in the treatment of hypertension (Patel et al. 1985). The meanings and role of drug treatments in the lay and professional spheres and their inter-relationships are thus subject to continuing processes of change, with an important aspect of this being the gradual adoption of the beliefs and practices associated with western medicine among ethnic groups whose own explanatory framework and treatments were derived from a differing cultural system.

References

Balarajan, R. 1991. Ethnic differences in mortality from ischaemic heart disease and cardiovascular disease in England and Wales. *British Medical Journal* **302**, 560–64.

Beecher, H. 1955. The powerful placebo. *Journal of the American Medical Association* **59**, 602–6.

Becker, M. H. 1985. Patient adherence to prescribed therapies. *Medical Care* **23**(5), 539–55.

Beevers, G. & M. Beevers 1993. Hypertension: impact on black and ethnic minority people. In *Access to health care for people from black and ethnic minorities*, A. Hopkins & V. Bahl (eds). London: Royal College of Physicians.

Bhopal, R. S. 1986. The inter-relationship of folk traditional and western medicine within an Asian community in Britain. *Social Science and Medicine* **22**(1), 99–105.

REFERENCES

Bledsoe, C. H. & M. Gaubaud 1985. The reinterpretation of western pharmaceuticals among the Mende of Sierra Leone. *Social Science and Medicine* 21(3), 275–82.

Blumhagen, D. 1980. Hyper-tension: a folk illness with a medical name. *Culture, Medicine and Psychiatry* 4, 197–227.

Chew, R. 1992. *Compendium of health statistics*, 8th edn. London: Office of Health Economics.

Conrad, P. 1985. The meaning of medications: another look at compliance. *Social Science and Medicine* 20, 29–37.

Cornwell, J. 1984. *Hard-earned lives: accounts of health and illness from East London*. London: Tavistock.

Davies, D. M. (ed.) 1981. *Textbook of adverse drug reactions*. Oxford: Oxford University Press.

Donovan, J. 1986. *We don't buy sickness, it just comes: deviance and reasoned decision-making?* London: Gower.

Donovan, J. & R. Blake 1992. Patient non-compliance: deviance or reasoned decision making. *Social Science and Medicine* 34(5), 507–13.

Eisenberg, L. 1977. Disease and illness: distinctions between professional and popular ideas of sickness. *Culture, Medicine and Psychiatry* 1(1), 9–23.

Fallsberg, M. 1991. *Reflections on medicines and medications: a qualitative analysis among people on long-term drug regimes*. Linköping: Linköping University.

Fletcher, A. E., P. J. Franks, C. J. Bulpitt 1988. The effect of withdrawing antihypertensive therapy: a review. *Journal of Hypertension* 6, 431-6.

Gabe, J. & N. Thorogood 1986. Prescribed drug use and the management of everyday life: the experiences of black and white working-class women. *Sociological Review* 34, 737–72.

Gabe, J., U. Gustafsson, M. Bury 1991. Mediating illness: newspaper coverage of tranquillizer dependence. *Sociology of Health and Illness* 13(3), 332–53.

Gilbert, A., N. Owen, C. Samon, J. M. Innes 1990. High levels of medication compliance and blood pressure control among hypertensives attending community pharmacies. *Journal of Social and Administrative Pharmacy* 7, 78–83.

Goulbourne, H. 1991. *Ethnicity and nationalism in post-imperial Britain*. Cambridge: Cambridge University Press.

Harwood, A. 1981. *Ethnicity and health care*. Cambridge, Mass.: Harvard University Press.

Hart, J. T. 1987. *Hypertension: community control of high blood pressure*. London: Churchill Livingstone.

Herskovits, M. J. 1948. *Man and his works*. New York: Knopf.

Hunt, L. M., B. Jordan, S. Irwin, C. H. Browner 1989. Compliance and the patients' perspective: controlling symptoms in everyday life. *Culture, Medicine and Psychiatry* 13, 315–34.

Illich, I. 1976. *Limits to medicine. Medical nemesis: the expropriation of health*. London: Marion Boyars.

Kleinman, A. 1980. *Patients and healers in the context of culture*. Berkeley: University of California Press.

Kwachi, I. & N. Wilson 1990. The evolution of anti-hypertensive therapy. *Social Science and Medicine* 31(11), 1239–43.

Medawar, C. 1992. *Power and dependence: social audit on the safety of medicines.* London: Social Audit Unit.

Meyer, D., H. Leventhal, M. Gutmann 1985. Common-sense models of illness: the example of hypertension. *Health Psychology* 4(2), 115–35.

Mitchell, M. F. 1983. Popular medical concepts in Jamaica and their impact on drug use. *The Western Journal of Medicine* 139(6), 841–7.

Montagne, M. 1988. The metaphorical nature of drugs and drug taking. *Social Science and Medicine* 26(4), 417–24.

Morgan, M. & C. Watkins 1988. Managing hypertension: beliefs and responses to medication among cultural groups. *Sociology of Health and Illness* 10, 561–78.

Patel, C. H., M. Mamot, D. J. Terry, M. Carruthers, B. Hunt, M. Patel 1985. Trial of relaxation in reducing coronary risk: four year follow up. *British Medical Journal* 290, 1103–6.

Roth, H. P. 1987. Ten year update on patient compliance research. *Patient Education and Counselling* 10, 107–16.

Sachs, L. & G. Tomson 1992. Medicines and culture – a double perspective on drug utilization in a developing country. *Social Science and Medicine* 34(3), 307–15.

Secretary of State for Health 1993. *The health of the nation: key area handbook: coronary heart disease and stroke.* London: Department of Health.

Sharma, U. M. 1990. Using alternative therapies: marginal medicine and central concerns. In *New directions in the sociology of health*, P. Abbott & G. Payne (eds). Basingstoke: Falmer.

Smaje, C. 1995. *Health, race and ethnicity: making sense of the evidence.* London: Kings Fund.

Sussman, L. K. 1988. The use of herbal and biomedical pharmaceuticals on Mauritius. In *The context of medicines in developing countries*. S. Van Der Geest & S. K. Whyte (eds), 199–215. Dordrecht: Kluwer.

Teague, A. 1993. *Ethnic group: first results from the 1991 census.* Population Trends No. 72. London: HMSO.

Thorogood, N. 1990. Caribbean home remedies and their importance for black women's health care in Britain. In *New directions in the sociology of health*, P. Abbott & G. Payne (eds), 140–52. Basingstoke: Falmer.

Part III

Chronic illness and modern medicine

Chapter 6

The critical moment: time, information and medical expertise in the experience of patients receiving coronary bypass surgery

Alan Radley

At the centre of this chapter is a paradox regarding patients' perspectives on the particular medical treatment offered; the surgical procedure that they undergo is not experienced directly by the individuals concerned. This is in spite of the fact that it is of key significance to them, both before and after their time in hospital. Patients anticipate receiving heart surgery, and they look back upon their recovery from it: but "it" – the operation itself – is, of necessity, beyond the horizon of their consciousness. This situation is not, of course, special to these kinds of patients or to this procedure. Nevertheless, to speak of the "experience of coronary bypass surgery" is always to refer to a time before the operation, and to a period after it has occurred. Having said that, the time of the operation itself, the procedures performed and the skills of the surgical team, are clearly of concern to the patients involved. The problem is that this is a "non-time" in their experience, the features of which must be inferred from what patients are told, and, subsequently, from their own bodily feelings. The paradox arises because this "non-time" will be/was (but in a sense, never is) a crucial moment in patients' lives, and the elaboration of this truth is linked inextricably to their views of medicine, its personnel and its practices.

The task of this chapter is to sketch out how this occurs, by means of reports given by a sample of male patients who were interviewed both before and after receiving this treatment. A brief overview of the operation is in order here. Coronary artery bypass graft surgery has today become a relatively common procedure in western medicine (English et al. 1984). It is used in cases where severe chest pain has not been relieved by a drug regime, and where X-ray examination of the heart and blood vessels shows a degree of arterial narrowing that warrants intervention to avoid an imminent heart attack. Briefly, the procedure involves taking a piece of vein (usually the saphenous vein from the leg), connecting it to the aorta, and then to a point on the affected coronary artery beyond the occluded section. In this way the narrowed part of the artery is bypassed, once more allowing blood to flow to the area of heart muscle that had been receiving an insufficient supply (Rapaport 1982). Within the medical profession, coronary bypass grafting is regarded by many cardiologists and surgeons as having become a relatively low-risk procedure offering the possibility of considerable angina relief to over 90 per cent of its recipients (Treasure 1983).

As will be explained below, this is the kind of description that patients are given, either when they are offered the treatment or when they come into hospital to receive it. There is a growing research literature that is concerned with the best ways to offer this information, to help patients prepare psychologically for the operation, and to aid in their recovery and rehabilitation in the weeks following treatment (Gillis 1984, Hochman 1982, Pimm & Feist 1984, Wilson-Barnett 1981). However, such recommendations and procedures are framed within aims set out from the perspective of medical staff. These aims necessitate "objective measures" to monitor and to guide the course of patient recovery. For that reason, they tell us little about how patients understand, evaluate and make use of what they are told by doctors, nurses and other personnel.

It is, of course, important to know how people in general think of operations such as heart transplants or coronary bypass surgery (Calnan & Williams 1992). However, there can be no generalizing from the person in a (broadly) healthy position, to someone who is told that a particular medical procedure is essential to his or her long, or even short-term survival. Coronary graft surgery is special within treatments for chronic diseases: it is a procedure that offers not only improvement in present health, but also the removal of the threat of sudden death in the near future. This chapter deals with this latter situation, which, though peculiar to a small group of individuals, can throw a special light upon the question of how lay perspectives on modern medicine are sharpened or developed.

Arguably, what patients "make of" medicine is important, both for their immediate participation in treatment and for their longer-term health behaviour. Certainly, it seems that a "poor" approach to surgery is detrimental to outcome (Bruce et al. 1983, Radley et al. 1987, Janis 1974). But what is meant by medicine in this context? Is it a sphere of ideas and practices experienced in a unitary fashion, away from other areas of one's life? And how are these ideas and practices apprehended – together or separately, formally or in more informal dealings with medical staff? There is good reason to bear in mind the point made by Bury (1982) (in the context of chronic illness) that medicine's role as a symbolic system facilitates, as well as constrains, people's actions and understanding during times of personal troubles and affliction. From that point of view, we should expect to find that individuals do not regard medicine as an "illegitimate reification", but as providing important and helpful "fixed points on a terrain of uncertainty". Extending this argument to the surgical treatment for heart disease, it is possible that medical knowledge plays a significant role in the lives of the individuals concerned, particularly as this is a time of potential anxiety and considerable uncertainty for them.

If this argument is sound, then medicine is not something evaluated at a distance, so to speak, but on occasions will be understood at a far more personal level. Receiving coronary bypass surgery is an example of this latter kind of occasion, when what should be understood is not just what people think of medicine, nor even the terms in which they think it. Instead, it is important to grasp how they come to comprehend it. This has implications for explaining the relationship between lay and medical ideas, which extend beyond the boundaries of the situation in which these particular patients find themselves.

Trust and threat in the anticipation of surgery

The project upon which this chapter is based was a prospective study of a cohort of 42 male patients and their wives (Radley 1988). The specific purpose of the study was to describe the different "adjustment styles" that the couples adopted in their everyday lives, and to relate these to measures of outcome. At the initial interview, when the men were offered surgery following angiographic investigation, data were collected about the couples' history of illness. A further interview was conducted with them at the time of admission for surgery, and then three times in the first 12 months after discharge from hospital. The main focus of the study was not, however, the couples' attitudes towards medicine, nor the men's experience of hospital treatment. We were more concerned with how they coped with the diagnosis and treatment of heart disease in the context of their lives at home. However, we did ask about the couples' views concerning the information given to them by medical staff, and particularly about their evaluation of the treatment in the light of the various ups and downs in the men's recovery. As well as this, there were many spontaneous expressions of feeling and opinion on the part of the couples concerning the doctors whom they met, the hospital where surgery took place, and the information provided at different times during the men's treatment.

Some of the patients had lived with heart disease for many years; others had only recently developed symptoms, sometimes following a heart attack. This meant that the experience of medicine, and of health professionals, varied across the sample. However, in all cases, the knowledge that they should now be treated by surgical means required a shift in their understanding of their condition and, by implication, in their relationship to medical practitioners. This shift was conveyed in their statements about the need for surgery, premised upon the (now perceived) seriousness of their condition:

> No, the heart itself apparently, the attack damaged my heart. Apparently it was a massive attack which I've only just realized. When I first had it, they told me it was a medium heart attack and I've always been led to believe that ever since till the surgeon told me yesterday that I'm in a really bad way.

> We both know I've got to have the operation. The surgeon in fact has talked more to the wife than he did to me, he's told her that if I don't have it done, that's it, so there's no feeling, "oh, I'll not have the operation", and carry on.

Surgery was perceived as necessary by (virtually) all of the men, and in many cases it was seen as life saving. This meant, as one of the more reluctant patients said, that it was "Hobson's choice" about whether or not to proceed with the operation. Right from the beginning, the knowledge that they "had to have the operation" and the promise that it would, at best, bring symptom relief, and at least, save their life, created for patients a special relationship with medicine. While breaking unwelcome news may be problematic for the doctor, the possibility of remedial treatment can be justified by reference to particular explanations of cause (e.g. "furring of the arteries") and the promise of control (Voysey 1972). This, then, legitimates the symptoms in terms of medical concepts, and can help to absolve the patients from feelings of responsibility for their condition. However, in the case of coronary artery disease, this absolution is conditional. Several of the men in this study spoke of the role of smoking and diet in the genesis of their condition. To the extent that they were, or had been smokers, this knowledge placed an onus on them to alter their behaviour if surgery was to be a success. That is, the diagnosis did not absolve them of all responsibility for their condition, and as a result, exerted greater power over their future intentions to comply with medical advice.

This process of legitimation depended upon an acceptance of the doctor's diagnosis. Where this was either unclear, or else did not square with the patient's own feelings, then a doubt remained that would be an important hindrance to the emergence of a relationship in which the patient could trust the outcome of the recommended surgical treatment. In a few cases, the diagnosis had been expressed in a way that puzzled and ultimately disturbed either the patient or his family:

Interviewer: What have you been told about the operation by the hospital?

Patient: That I'm not very pleased with. I went Tuesday and they told me and my wife it could be touch and go if I even come through it because I've got a heart disease.

Interviewer: You knew that before?

Patient: I didn't know, no. It puts you off a bit.

Interviewer: Has that made you think twice about whether you want it doing?

Patient: No, I still want it doing, but I wish they hadn't told me. My doctor he played hell about it. He said they [the doctors at the hospital] shouldn't have told you at all.

This man's wife was also confused and angry. She said:

Our doctor, he don't know nothing about it . . . He says as far as he's concerned all he knows he's got to have that bypass. We know that. What is this bloody diseased heart?

These comments show the uncertainty engendered in the patient (and family) by a diagnosis that was not accepted, perhaps because it was at variance with what they had previously understood. This understanding also came from the patient's own way of coming to terms with the symptoms of coronary disease, and its implications. What has been called the need to "complete" the knowledge gained from specialist sources is here frustrated by the perceived inconsistency of present and past diagnoses of the patient's condition (Bury 1982).

Where this inconsistency occurred, it raised questions about the doctor's competence, which could generalize to a distrust of how the patient was being managed in the wider sphere. Where this included the anticipated operation itself, then the patient was faced with considerable doubt and anxiety about the wisdom of proceeding with the recommended treatment. This was dissipated to some degree by the knowledge that medical technology allowed the doctors to "see" the condition in ways denied to the patient. One man who did not suffer greatly from angina or shortness of breath, and hence did not (literally) feel the need for surgery, said:

It's probably serious medically more than its appearance. I've had tests and know what's wrong with me, so it's got to be better than having something and you don't know. I'm in the right place to find out what is the problem and I do know now.

For the majority (and ultimately for all) of the patients in the sample, there was an acceptance of the necessity that they undergo bypass surgery to relieve their condition. This acceptance was not, however, an easy one, nor was it something that happened in a single moment. Instead, the willingness to undergo surgery involved taking on an existential dilemma, concerning, on the one hand, the promise of symptom relief, and on the other, the prospect of pain and the possibility of death (Radley et al. 1987). This dilemma was something that was mulled over by many of the men, and their families, for the whole period between angiography and admission. It involved, as a key part to its resolution, fashioning an image of medical practitioners (particularly the surgeons) as authorities in their field and as experts in their practice.

The threat of surgery appeared in several different forms, although direct references to dying in the operation were expressed by relatively few patients. This did not mean, however, that the operation itself was of little concern to the men once they had accepted its inevitability. References to "bad nights" and "poor concentration", as well as other comments from wives, showed that a procedure that would not be experienced (in the sense of "known directly") was sometimes thoroughly examined in anticipation. One man, unusually forthright, put it as follows:

> Well, I'm frightened to death. That is the main feeling. I try not to harp on it too much. I find my worst time is at night because I can't remember the last time I had a good night's sleep. Sometime during the night I wake up anyway and subconsciously, I don't know. I'm just hoping they do something. The only thing I can think about now is everybody says how good it will be taking me down there, doing the operation, and afterwards; I think it's just the point of the afterwards. I'm just hoping that I wake up and see the right sort of angels.

Not all patients were concerned solely about surviving the operation on their heart. For some it was the efficacy of the anaesthetic that mattered most to them, and the possibility that they might, through an accident, be conscious during the procedure. As one man said:

> Not the operation itself, because it doesn't concern me that, it's got nothing to do with me what they do inside there, it's how they put you to sleep.

These various fears and worries about the operation were discussed by some patients and wives, and not at all by others. In nearly every case, however, there was evidence that the prospect of the husbands' surgery was of great concern to the wives, and in some cases had been the cause of their seeking help for symptoms from their family doctor. There was evidence that they, too, continued to vacillate about the need for their husbands to undergo surgery:

> Interviewer: How much do you feel you both want the operation?
>
> Wife: It's a difficult question. At the moment 100 per cent. If you ask me in half an hour I might tell you I don't want him to have it at all.

Bypass surgery contained, therefore, a double prospect; on the one hand, symptom relief (if not "cure"), and on the other, the possibility of pain and death. The anxiety attaching to this was amplified by the fact that the decision to have surgery was, in the last analysis, made by the patient himself, together with his family. The burden of this decision was partly offset by patients emphasizing that the need for surgery had been spelled out by the doctors, the experts who "know best".

The anxiety and fear relating to surgery were handled in two particular ways, each leading towards a special relationship of the patient to medical staff. Anxiety about the procedure was minimized by patients deliberately restricting information about the procedure itself. Having first mulled over what might happen in surgery, several patients then distanced the operation from themselves by accepting it as a period of non-time, of non-being. This was consistent with the idea that it was futile to think oneself into it, to contemplate oneself as a body lying on the table, waiting to be cut open:

> They have described the operation to me, given me opportunities to ask questions and I found talking to neighbours who have had the operation very helpful. They've really told me more but, in fairness, the hospital did say "what do you want to know?" . . . I'm happy, I don't want to bury my head in the sand but I don't want to know all of it.
>
> Mr C. [the surgeon] told me nearly everything without going into the technical details which only a doctor understands. He told me what he would have to do, where he was taking the arteries from and where he was putting them. That's as much as I know, as much as I need to know.

However, the main antidote to the fear of surgery was an investment by the patients in the skills of the doctors. They focused either upon the competence of the surgeons in particular, or upon the helpfulness of medical staff in general, who were seen as having put the patient at his ease. Emphasizing the surgeon's skills (even if these could not be appraised, even indirectly) meant that the men could put their trust in medicine. This trust reflected a particular relationship to doctors and nursing staff, in which the patient placed himself (i.e. his life) entirely in their hands. He had faith that they would bring to bear an expertise and care justifying his decision to proceed. This had the effect of removing from the patient the worry about whether he was making the right choice, for it was this particular burden (electing for surgery) that disturbed many of the families to whom we spoke. Here are some examples reflecting this attitude.

> Last Tuesday I saw Dr E. [the cardiologist]. He asked me a lot of questions and he said that he would see me again before the operation. I saw Mr S. [the surgeon] and he said that the other two doctors had declined doing my operation as it was a high risk . . . but that he is going to do it. And he said, "you've no need to worry whatsoever, it is my worry not yours". He explained what was going to happen.

> I'm not worried about it or anything like that. I'm in professional hands, like. When you've got something wrong with your car you take it to the professionals, don't you?

> In fact, I think it's the best hospital I've ever been into . . . there they tell you everything and exactly what they are going to do and they meet you and talk to you. I think it's a smashing place, I do. (Wife) The surgeon, he gives you confidence. I don't know whether it's just that particular man, but after we came out you felt as though you were really leaving it up to him, and you could leave it up to him for everything being all right.

With the adoption of this kind of attitude, patients could keep their fears and anxieties in check. That is, the faith placed in the medical staff, particularly the surgeon who would carry out the procedure, was, in part, a product of the need to come to terms with the threats that surgery held. It appeared to be a more specific, and more urgent expression of what has been termed the "theodicy" relating individuals to the symbolic universe of modern medicine (Voysey 1975). Whatever the couples had thought about medicine in general prior to the consultation leading to the offer of bypass surgery, now it was the particulars of "these doctors" and "this hospital" that concerned them.

This expression of faith was neither a simple outcome nor one common to all of the patients and spouses in the sample. Some couples were more successful than others in conveying a sense of having come to terms with the need for surgery and with its risks. The wives were more outspoken than their husbands about the mental toll taken by the length of time waiting to hear of an admission date (anything from 1 to 21 months). It seemed that what might be termed "blind faith" in the medical staff was expressed more by patients who were most anxious, who needed to amplify the skills of the surgeon and the reputation of the hospital in order to stave off the fear that they would die during the operation.

Once assimilated by patients and spouses, medical knowledge seemed to have two functions. It provided an authoritative view of the patient's condition, such that the recommendation of surgery seemed to follow "naturally" (or at least, sensibly) from the diagnosis of his condition. As part of this, the technology of modern medicine that allowed the cardiologists and surgeons to look into the patient's heart and blood vessels gave them a privileged perspective that had to be taken at face value. Therefore, on the one hand, medical knowledge framed the patients' experience and symptoms in a way that displaced other, competing explanations for what might be the cause of their physical condition. (For examples of these, see Radley 1988.) It also helped to normalize events (such as bouts of chest pain) that were potentially frightening, by making these into things "you've got to expect when you are waiting for an operation", as one couple were told by their GP.

The second function of medical knowledge was to suspend the patient's claim, or need to imagine, inquire into or otherwise elaborate upon the operation itself. Mention has already been made of the many statements by patients that "they knew all they needed to know" about the operation. This meant that, when we spoke to the couples near the time of the men's admission to hospital, we were often told that they did not speak about the impending surgery to other people, and sometimes little to each other. As was noted in a study of a family where the father waited for just this operation:

> Anxieties, fears, terrors and concerns cannot surface or become contagious because they are safeguarded by the collective resolve not to air differences, nuances of doubt, and the corresponding resolve to give ground to another effortlessly, without contest, dispute or voiced reservation. The [family] stays together in the same field by getting out of each other's way (Bermann 1973: 82).

The couples' trust in the doctors helped to make this waiting bearable. It also had the effect of sealing off the operation in time, making it an event that, though not to be explored or discussed for itself, transformed all other activity that would lead up to it. Though medical issues might not be at the forefront of everyday conversation, they were forever in the background, because all of life now waited upon the news of an admission date and the inevitable outcome of surgery.

Prior to the operation, the patients had built up a view of medicine and of doctors that was grounded in their coming to terms with this life-saving, but potentially life-threatening procedure. How they thought about medical staff was not something that could be explained only in terms of distinct and separate meetings or happenings. Discrete events did matter (such as the postponing of surgery at the last moment), but always in the context of the relationship that patients had adopted with respect to medicine and its expertise. The giving-over of responsibility for the patients' life to another person (someone who will open one's chest, take and modify one's heart), rendered the "non-time" of the operation into something special. In consequence, this had the effect of permeating all of the patients' actions that led up to this episode.

This can be considered to be an example of "narrative reconstruction" (Williams 1984), in which the breaking of the assumed links between life's mundane events requires the individual to re-establish the connections between body, self and society. In the case of some of the patients awaiting surgery, this meant more than just revising their biographies: it meant living them in a different way. Through the ways that they anticipated events, reaching out for some things, avoiding others, the men did not simply respond to a ready-made world, but were active in fashioning an approach to surgery in which they, themselves, appeared coherent and morally creditable individuals. While it may be true to say, following Collingwood (quoted in Williams 1984), that "every present has a past of its own", for these couples their present was given its specific form through the anticipation of a particular future. That anticipation was, quite literally, lived out by them. This meant that the impact of medicine lay beyond changes in what patients knew or said: it impacted on how they, and their spouses, lived their lives, on how they oriented themselves toward any and every aspect of their daily existence (Radley 1993).

The dominant position of medical thinking, as adopted by patient and spouse, provided both a beginning (cause) and an end (surgery) to the temporal present in which the couples lived their lives. While this was always apparent in the period prior to the men's admission, it was also of importance in the weeks and months following surgery. The way that they would come to think of doctors and medicine immediately after the operation was actually more striking. However, it owed much to the way that the men (and their wives) had come to terms with these matters in the period prior to undergoing the operation.

Fantastic! Patients' views of medical staff after surgery

It is, perhaps, not surprising to hear patients who have undergone heart surgery express their gratitude to the medical staff who treated and cared for them. In the previous section it was pointed out that coronary bypass grafting, though generally a safe procedure (at the time of the study the mortality rate was of the order of 3 per cent), still involves risks. These risks are minimized by the skills of the surgical team, so that patients are grateful not only for the symptom relief that the procedure aims at, but for their safe passage through the operation itself. While not every patient in this study felt that the operation had been a technical success (there were one or two exceptions), none expressed other than positive sentiments about the staff and the hospital where they had been treated. These are typical comments made at interview four months after the operation:

> Well, to be honest, the medical staff at [the hospital] they are just out of this world. I've never been to another hospital like it. I know the hospital itself is not all it should be but that's not their fault, the staff are magnificent. Right from top to bottom because they are just like a big family. They are not like any other medical staff I've ever met before.

> Really, the medical staff is the [most helpful], definitely. They looked after you marvellously after the operation. Dr H., he just told me I looked well, and said, "you are going on fine". There's nothing else he can do really.

One wife said:

> I'd just like to say that the treatment at the hospital was absolutely marvellous, and the experience of going into the intensive care ward was an eye-opener for me. I was a bit apprehensive about it but I didn't stay, I just went in to see that he was all right; and it was wonderful and everybody was hovering round and working all the machines, I came home thinking things were going to be all right.

The view of medicine in the above comment about staff "working all the machines" reveals the dramatic or presentational aspect to the hospital experience. In Goffman's (1959) terms, such technology is a "prop" to the selves that medical staff fashion in the course of playing their professional roles. As it is employed during the preparation of patients for surgery, and in the period of intensive care afterwards, this technology can become extraordinarily significant for the patients, even if they only dimly comprehend its specific functions. Perhaps for that reason, the mystique surrounding equipment becomes attached to the staff themselves, confirming the theodicy of the patient in respect to medicine, and more particularly their faith in the skills of the doctors and nursing staff.

Even where the outcome of surgery had not been as successful as was hoped for, it was rare for any hint of blame to be attached to medical staff. As one patient with little symptom relief said, "they've got to try". One wife of a man who had been left with other, quite discomforting, problems as a result of surgery, said that she saw the outcome of the operation as "a disappointment". However, on being asked whether she could do with more information from the hospital at that stage of her husband's recovery, she said:

I wouldn't criticize [the hospital] in any way, shape or form.

The patients and their families retained this feeling of gratitude towards staff and hospital over the period of 12 months following the operation. It was even typical of patients who, sometimes months after discharge, found that they had a return of the chest pains that the operation was intended to remove. Clearly, their attitudes to the medical staff did not hinge solely upon the specific outcome of the operation, but also upon their experience of their time in hospital. This time included both the period of nursing care in the two days prior to the operation, and the seven to ten days after surgery. Where, as pointed out above, the period of care involved face-to-face contact with nurses, and a series of recoverable experiences, the operation itself inevitably remained beyond the patients' immediate experience. This meant that it was not recoverable directly, so that its significance had to be established in an indirect way. How this mattered for the patients' views of medicine, and what it had done for them, will be discussed in the remainder of this section.

The feeling of trust that had been established previously was no longer so obvious, in the way that it had been prior to the time of the operation. However, it had created a relationship of patient to doctor (and nurse) that proved to be critical in the way that many of the men reoriented themselves after surgery. In effect, surgery was seen by many as having been a special kind of ordeal or passage that they, with the help of medical staff, had endured. The trust that had been given had been repaid in a general sense of having "come through as a person", not just in the specific outcome of relief of symptoms.

The comments provided at the beginning of this section are a testimony to this situation. However, they did not provide the most revealing evidence of how the couples (particularly the patients) were thinking about the medical treatment received. This came, unexpectedly, in small criticisms of the hospital and follow-up experience. For example, there were several comments about how couples wished that more information had been given prior to the operation. (This was at odds with statements made at the time that they "only wanted to know so much"). It was as if, having isolated the impending operation with all its uncertainties, once it had been passed through successfully, individuals wanted to know more about it. One wife made this comment:

> I thought afterwards, why didn't I ask? There was a health visitor there, why didn't I ask her a little bit more about what it was going to be like when he came out, because it was rather a shock.

One reason for couples expressing dissatisfaction with the information given, was that they wanted to be able to understand and not worry about unexpected hiccoughs in the men's recovery. In part, this also appeared to be because they wanted to know that they were making a "normal" recovery, and wished to avoid drawing attention to their situation as one requiring special attention. Later on, at the one-year post-surgery interview, this need for information would be generalized to an argument that patients could have obtained useful information from individuals who had received the operation earlier on. This would not only have allowed a degree of predictability, but would also have provided normative guidelines for how a "bypass patient" is expected to feel, and expected to behave. (One patient who had experienced hallucinations on the ward after surgery, and believed he had been quite unco-operative with the nursing staff, was afterwards faced with having to try and account for his behaviour in ways that could minimize his deviant status.)

Subsequent visits for check-ups in the months after surgery gave opportunities for patients to meet medical staff and to communicate their feelings about the operation's success (or, in a few cases, its qualified failure). These meetings were considered to be quite important, because they were also opportunities for the men and their wives to establish "how the operation had gone". In a few cases, there were doubts among patients about how many grafts had actually been placed. There were also questions about the long-term state of their heart, and others concerning the improvement in life-quality that, the men had been told, the operation could offer. Not surprisingly, where patients could not resolve these questions satisfactorily, nor (and this was equally important) re-establish themselves in relation to the surgeon after the treatment was over, there emerged a sense of disappointment.

The only [question] I did ask – the doctor the other week when I went – I should have seen Dr E. and I saw his assistant, a lady doctor, and she did go through my notes because before the operation, Mr C. who did the operation, told me he was making three repairs . . . after I came out of intensive care, he said I've only put in two. I still don't exactly know although the lady doctor at [the hospital] the other week said . . .

Yes, really. I went through the hospital in about eight days, which seemed to me to be very quick. I was glad that I was able to come out at the time but then apart from going for pricks for blood tests I didn't hear. The appointment was quite a long way away from coming out and then, when I did go to the appointment, I didn't see one of the surgeons or perhaps one of the people that assisted, but a relatively junior doctor. And I just thought, it would have wrapped it up so much nicer if one had seen somebody who had actually, perhaps, been present and part of the team. Perhaps he was.

The surgeon I saw later on was one of the surgeons that worked under Mr C. I never did see [him], only once when I went for an interview for him to explain what it was all about. I never ever saw him from that day to this. Yet he is supposedly the consultant surgeon that I saw but I never saw him again. Not even walking about the ward, I didn't even see him.

This wish to have had more information about the procedure and the course of recovery, together with the need to see the surgeon who carried out one's operation, were part of a process of recovering the operation in a new way. This latter kind of "recovery" involved a working-through of the time when the patient was in intensive care, and on the ward afterwards. It also involved, crucially, a kind of psychological re-admission of the "non-time" of the operation into a central portion of their life. The significance of this experience was not easy for the patients to express, and no quotation from the transcripts can do justice to the feeling to which many of them referred. However, this feeling did remain over the course of time in which they had been treated. That many patients felt they remained "in the debt" of the surgeons was still evident one year after their operation. There were several references by patients to the need "not to undo the good work that they have done for me", underlining once more how the putative relationship with staff legitimated the patients' position.

One other feature of the patients' memory of their time in hospital was the sense of camaraderie that several of them expressed. This related, once more, to the feeling that they had gone through something special together. Though they were alone in the hours of their own operation, in the ward and in the weeks afterwards, they shared their experiences together. The critical time of the operation effectively gained in significance through being a common "non-experience", if it can be put that way. Sometimes the significance of that sharing came, as with other comments, through what appeared as criticism. In his final interview, one year after surgery, one man said:

> You think you're on your own, you think you're the only one and nobody understands what you're going through. They know the physical problems, but nobody seems to care about how you are thinking . . . Yes, you do worry, you can't not. No, you look round to try and talk to someone. Talking does help. After the operation we used to talk, and everybody used to say – "if we had talked about this before". You've got something to look forward to which makes a difference. You're more open. When you've had it done people start talking.

The sharing of the hospital experience can be considered to be an example of collective memory (Middleton & Edwards 1990), that captures not only the feelings of the time, but also confirms the debt that is felt to be owed by patients to the doctors and nurses who treated and cared for them. As already mentioned, these feelings were often regarded as private by the patients themselves, and not easily spoken of openly. To illustrate this, it was left to the wife of one patient at the eight-month interview to tell us that her husband had daily telephone contact with another patient, with whom he had spent his stay in hospital. On a larger scale, the establishment of a self-help group offering support to past patients, and counselling to current ones, was founded on just such common feeling (Simpson 1993). It is also noteworthy that among its main tasks were (and continue to be) to raise money for equipment for the cardiac wards, to invite speakers from the world of medical research, and to keep ex-patients in close touch with the staff of the hospital where they received their treatment.

Marks on one's biography: implications for the evaluation of medicine

What is one to make of the positive reports given by these patients and their spouses, and of the gratitude shown to the nursing and medical staff who cared for them? Are they exceptional in the context of surgery in general, and are they indicative of a wide acceptance of the power and authority of medicine among the British general public? No claim is made here that the reports given by these couples are typical of surgery patients in general. Also, the particularly dramatic form of surgical intervention in coronary artery disease means that their experience is not likely to be shared by individuals afflicted by many other chronic diseases.

In spite of these caveats, it is important to note that positive reports by patients appear often in the literature about the experience of heart surgery. Prior to the widespread use of coronary grafting, a study of patients who had undergone heart operations to correct valve or septal defects found that their most pleasant recollection was "the attitude of dedicated concern shown by the doctors and nurses" (Blachly & Blachly 1968: 529). It is important to note that this "dedicated concern" was not limited to specific procedures or the giving of information, but was attributed by patients to the staff members themselves.

One explanation for such a positive appraisal concerns the patient's commitment to what is regarded as a discomforting, life-threatening and medically elaborate procedure. This results in their experiencing a large measure of "cognitive dissonance" (Nixon 1980). This argument maintains that the patient's (and, one should add, the spouse/partner's) considerable investment in surgery demands, subsequently, that they feel the operation to have worked. This outcome has been demonstrated even in cases where patients have experienced post-operation pain, delirium and a poor surgical result (Frank et al. 1972).

Such a situation is not very different from the proposition that coronary bypass surgery works because of a "placebo effect" (Moerman 1983). Evidence for this comes from studies that have found that symptomatic improvement can occur regardless of the completeness of revascularization, which is the aim of the procedure (Valdes et al. 1979). Recognizing this possibility, cardiologists and cardio-thoracic surgeons have been keen to point out that the placebo effect cannot alone account for the "physiologic benefit" of coronary grafting that other studies have been able to demonstrate (Rapaport 1982, Treasure 1990).

Taken together, the patient's undoubted investment in the operation, and the commitment of medical staff to its benefits, point to their joint involvement in an ideology articulated through medical practice (Price 1984). In the case of coronary grafting, this is specific in its use of "plumbing" metaphors to do with the blocking and unblocking of arteries. It also shares certain features with surgery in general in its parallel with the repairing, rebuilding or remodelling of machines (Bates 1990). However, the belief in the technological power of modern medicine is insufficient by itself to account for patients' beliefs in the healing powers of medical personnel.

It is in the patient's passage through the surgical procedure that this existential commitment is to be found. While the discourse of doctors is clearly important in establishing the authority of medicine (Fox 1992), this alone cannot explain the experience of the individuals interviewed in this study. As Blachly & Blachly (1968) point out, it was the actions of the staff rather than their words that conveyed this positive attitude, "this infusion of hope", most indelibly.

One way of accounting for this is to see the patient's passage as a transformation of a kind similar to that encountered in studies of religious experience. The healing powers of the medical staff extend beyond their technical skills and the material changes that they are able to bring about to the patient's body. The sphere of these powers is not a material but an existential one. They are brought to bear upon doubts and fears that concern matters of life and death. In the case of the cardiac surgery patient, these matters can throw into doubt many of the taken-for-granted ideas that bring comfort and assurance to everyday life. The healing powers of medicine lie in bringing about an ordering of, a meaning within experiences that, at their best, are inchoate, and, at their worst, revolve about a hollow of angst. This ordering takes place because the patient believes in the surgeon's and the nurses' commitment to care in general, and to his or her wellbeing specifically.

Calling this a "placebo effect" does less than justice to what is being proposed. It suggests, unwisely, a contrast between the material and the existential spheres, as if what happens "psychologically" might be judged separately from (and either better or worse than) what is done "physically" to the patient. In fact, it is knowledge of the surgeon's intrusion into the material aspect of the body – diverting the patient's lifeblood and incising the heart – that reflects the potential for transformation of the patient's life situation. The operation is, in this sense, a drama, a realm of significant meaning, in its evocation of powers that are irreducible to the cuttings and sewings involved. To take the "plumbing" metaphor literally is to mistake this rhetorical device for a "mere metaphor", i.e. to take it as the reason why patients are grateful to the surgeon. To ignore it, in the course of elevating the placebo effect above practice, is to make an error of a different kind. Then it seems that belief or ideology by itself is operating, somehow above and beyond the material features of surgery.

Instead, I would like to turn, once more, to a consideration of coronary bypass surgery as a moment, both in the sense of an instant in time and as a point about which other events turn, a kind of liminoid period (Turner 1982). It is a critical period, which at once disrupts the person's life, and yet is presented (by doctors) as the only route to a healthier existence. It is also a psychological and social turning point in the life of the patient and spouse, in that it ties together body, self and personal world to form a parameter about which biographical reconstruction must take place.

I have already made a case for seeing the operation itself as central to this process, in spite of it being a time of non-experience. References to the ways in which patients actively went over their time in hospital, linking up experiences, asking about details of the surgical procedure, comparing their behaviour to that of other patients – all these things testify to an accommodation, an incorporation of medicine within their lives. At one level, therefore, the way that surgeons and nurses were seen as "marvellous" derives from this quite elaborate, and often joint reconstruction of what happened to them during their time in hospital. The medical knowledge that had so structured and limited thought prior to the operation, became the subject of those very personal and social concerns that it had effectively contained (and protected) beforehand.

However, this view still makes it seem that doctors, nurses and physiotherapists were simply re-evaluated in the light of the way that they appeared to the patient in the weeks and months after surgery; that is, as if they had changed as objects of the patient's consideration. Arguably, the reconstructions of the time in hospital are better understood if we think of the change as having occurred to the *relationship* between patient and medical staff. Medicine (as represented by what had been done to the patient) had become incorporated into the person's biography. Coronary bypass surgery was not something that the patients remembered, or judged, as one might remember or judge a person who was met on a train. Instead, *being a bypass patient* – having passed through that non-experience – had established a place *from which* to reconstruct one's view of life. For many of these patients, medicine was not simply an object of consideration but was part of their identity, their heritage – a mark on their biography.

This incorporation of medicine into patients' biographies took place at many levels during the hospital experience. Mention has already been made of specific meetings with doctors, of the care of nursing staff and the role of advanced technology. In the remembering of their passage through this life-threatening/life-saving experience, many of these separate events were run together in a narrative that was located in time and space. That space was the hospital itself, which, for many of the men, took on a special "character". That character was key in the formation and operation of the self-help group that ex-patients organized to counsel and advise new and past bypass surgery patients (Simpson 1993). It was kept alive in the conversations and reminiscences of the group's members about their time in hospital, underlining both a common experience that they had "come through", and a significant identity that they shared as patients in relation to those medical staff at that hospital. Recently, the hospital in question has been closed and its cardiac facilities moved to a new hospital nearby. In spite of the promise of better facilities, one ex-patient was explicit in locating the powers that he believed are conducive to healing, in the broadest sense of the term:

We all feel scared of what will happen when Groby Road Hospital closes. I just feel that Link-up [the support group] is GRH, and GRH is Link-up. Glenfield hasn't got the same magic. It deals with other things. Can you detach Link-up [from GRH] and keep it all there? (Simpson 1993: 81).

Such deep memories of personally significant events (see the allusion in the above quote to "magic") are not confined to experiences of medicine and surgery. They are also the stuff of tragedies and of horrors, as well as of times of impenetrable joy. In this context, they gave shape to feelings that were not always coherently expressed by the individuals in our sample, but were always tangibly there nonetheless. The point to be taken is that one does not just "have" a perspective on medicine, or just "have" opinions about doctors or nurses. These perspectives must be gained and modified in some way, and the manner in which this happens is a key feature of how they are later communicated and understood.

It might be that much of what has been discussed above is applicable to any serious operation, or to any medical procedure thought to be critical or potentially dangerous. The notion of the "non-experience" is relevant to such situations, with its implications for the restructuring of personal time and space. Directly pertinent to this chapter is the question, "what does this tell us about how people regard medicine, and doctors?" The answer must be that it shows that patients are not only judges (or conceptualizers) who perceive medical staff, their procedures or their places of work as objects at a distance from themselves. It is because patients are also *embodied* beings, who in this case have submitted themselves to surgery and intensive care, that their basis of judgement has been changed. In a significant sense, the surgeons and nurses are now "part of them" in a way that eludes the empirical methods commonly employed within social and psychological science. However, even if we cannot address these questions in precise terms, they nevertheless speak volumes about the capacity for modern medicine to be incorporated into people's lives, as well as to reach inside their bodies.

References

Bates, M. S. 1990. A critical perspective on coronary artery disease and coronary bypass surgery. *Social Science and Medicine* 30, 249–60.

Bermann, E. 1973. Regrouping for survival: approaching dread and three phases of family interaction. *Journal of Comparative and Family Studies* 4, 63–87.

Blachly, P. H. & B. J. Blachly 1968. Vocational and emotional status of 263 patients after heart surgery. *Circulation* 38, 524–32.

REFERENCES

Bruce, E. H., R. A. Bruce, K. F. Hossack, F. Kusumi 1983. Psychosocial coping strategies and cardiac capacity before and after coronary artery bypass surgery. *International Journal of Psychiatry in Medicine* **13**, 69–84.

Bury, M. 1982. Chronic illness as biographical disruption. *Sociology of Health and Illness* **4**, 167–82.

Calnan, M. & S. Williams 1992. Images of scientific medicine. *Sociology of Health and Illness* **14**, 233–54.

English, T. A. H., A. R.Bailey, J. F. Dark, W. G. Williams 1984. The UK cardiac surgical register, 1977–82. *British Medical Journal* **289**, 1205–8.

Fox, N. J. 1992. *The social meaning of surgery.* Milton Keynes: Open University Press.

Frank, K. A., S. S. Heller, D. S. Kornfeld 1972. A survey of adjustment to cardiac surgery. *Archives of Internal Medicine* **130**, 735–8.

Gillis, C. L. 1984. Reducing family stress during and after coronary artery bypass surgery. *Nursing Clinics of North America* **19**, 103–12.

Goffman, E. 1959. *The presentation of self in everyday life.* New York: Anchor Books.

Hochman, G. 1982. *Heart bypass: what every patient should know.* New York: St Martin's Press.

Janis, I. 1974. *Psychological stress: psychoanalytic and behavioral studies in surgical patients.* New York: Academic Press.

Middleton, D. & D. Edwards (eds) 1990. *Collective remembering.* London: Sage.

Moerman, D. E. 1983. Physiology and symbols: the anthropological implications of the placebo effect. In *The anthropology of medicine: from culture to method*, 2nd edn. L. Romanucci-Ross, D. E. Moerman, L. R. Tancredi (eds). New York: Bergin & Garvey.

Nixon, P. G. F. 1980. Effects of medical vs surgical treatment on symptoms in stable angina pectoris. *Circulation* **61**, 1269.

Pimm, J. P. & J. Feist 1984. *Psychological risks of coronary bypass surgery.* New York: Plenum.

Price, L. 1984. Art, science, faith and medicine: the implications of the placebo effect. *Sociology of Health and Illness* **6**, 61–73.

Radley, A. 1988. *Prospects of heart surgery: psychological adjustment to coronary bypass grafting.* New York: Springer-Verlag.

Radley, A. 1993. The role of metaphor in adjustment to chronic illness. In *Worlds of illness: biographical and cultural perspectives on health and disease*, A. Radley (ed.), 109–23. London: Routledge.

Radley, A., R. Green, M. Radley 1987. Impending surgery: the expectations of male coronary patients and their wives. *International Rehabilitation Medicine* **8**, 154–61.

Rapaport, E. 1982. An overview of issues. Technology assessment forum on coronary artery bypass surgery. *Circulation* **66** (Supplement III), 3–5.

Simpson, R. 1993. *Self-help groups. The role and function of mutual support: case study of "Link-up" – a support group for pre- and post-operative cardiac patients.* Unpublished MA thesis, Loughborough University, UK.

Treasure, T. 1983. Coronary artery bypass surgery. *British Journal of Hospital Medicine* **30**, 259–63.

Treasure, T. 1990. Coronary surgery: an update. *British Journal of Hospital Medicine* **43**, 459–63.

Turner, V. 1982. *From ritual to theatre: the human seriousness of play*. New York: Performing Arts Journal Publications.

Valdes, M., B. D. McCallister, D. R. McConahay, W. A. Reed, D. A. Killen, M. Arnold 1979. "Sham operation" revisited: a comparison of complete vs unsuccessful coronary artery bypass. *American Journal of Cardiology* **43**, 382.

Voysey, M. 1972. Official agents and the legitimation of suffering. *Sociological Review* **20**, 533–51.

Voysey, M. 1975. *A constant burden: the reconstitution of family life*. London: Routledge & Kegan Paul.

Williams, G. 1984. The genesis of chronic illness: narrative reconstruction. *Sociology of Health and Illness* **6**, 174–200.

Wilson-Barnett, J. 1981. Assessment of recovery: with special reference to a study of post-operative cardiac patients. *Journal of Advanced Nursing* **6**, 435–45.

Chapter 7

Narratives of normality: end-stage renal-failure patients' experience of their transplant options

Uta Gerhardt

The medical, sociological and sociolinguistic problem

End-stage renal failure may be treated by two equally efficient treatment modes, namely dialysis and transplantation. Dialysis treatment is based on the principle of purifying the blood or peritoneal fluids through a machine or mechanical device extracting toxic substances from the body. Transplant treatment, however, is based on the principle of implanting a functioning graft into the patient's body.

The transplanted organ is positioned in the lower left abdominal cavity while the patient's own diseased kidneys are either left where they are to fulfil rudimentary metabolic functions, or the patient is nephrectomized which is often medically advisable. In either case, the patient's kidney function is taken over by the transplanted graft. It prevents uraemia, the deadly condition of inadvertent self-poisoning brought about through the body's metabolic waste. In this vein, the renal transplant secures the prolongation of life of the end-stage renal-failure patient for a time span that is known to have exceeded 20 years. Since transplantation surgery was only introduced in the 1960s, the time span of longevity added through a transplant operation may in future improve even further. Since the 1960s, dramatic improvements of surgical techniques as well as of immuno-suppressive drugs have raised the success rate of renal transplantation considerably. Sequential transplants are possible and have been given in tens of thousands of cases. If a transplant fails, which is not uncommon, the "gift of life" (Fox & Swazey 1974, Simmons et al. 1977) may be repeated but only, at most, five times (Challand 1972).

As for the origin of kidney transplants, two options are open. First the organ may be donated by a relative who gives one of his or her kidneys to a patient who otherwise would die, or would have to resort to a choice between the other treatment modes that are deemed less desirable in terms of re-acquiring normality. These are cadaver-donor transplantation, or long-term dialysis treatment. Alternatively, the patient receives a kidney from an anonymous donor. The latter is often a victim of a traffic accident who, due to brain damage, has no chance of survival and whose relatives agree to have the kidneys removed for transplantation. Although both modes of renal transplant therapy allow for better re-normalization than dialysis treatment, live-donor transplants and cadaver-donor transplants are not equivalent in their value for the patient.

Since live-donor transplant donors are first-degree relatives, their tissue matches that of the patient often so closely that only a minimum of immunosuppressive drugs may be needed to prevent rejection of the graft immediately after the operation but also on a long-term basis. Lower dosage of immunosuppressants, to be sure, diminishes such frequent side-effects as severe osteoporosis, or gross weight changes (up to 50 pounds) due to retention of water in the body tissues caused by steroid medication. In contrast, cadaver-donor transplantation is less advantageous. Whereas tissue-typing is also performed between donors and recipients of cadaver-donor transplants, their compatibility may be less; this means that higher doses of immunosuppressive medication may be needed and generally the risk of transplant failure is higher.

The risk of failure, it must be remembered, never goes away completely, although it diminishes over time (for a variable time period). Once a patient has survived the operation, rejection of the graft is dangerously likely during the first 6–9 months after transplantation, but after this a functioning transplant *may* work for years and maybe decades. Rejection of a grafted organ has a number of reasons. It may be due to the nature of the patient's renal disease (e.g. when cysts are the causal agent of the kidney failure), or to the quality of the organ (e.g. when a relatively long time span has elapsed between explantation and implantation of the graft), medication (i.e. some immunosuppressive drugs such as Cyclosporin A are themselves nephrotoxic), or a wide array of other circumstances that may or may not be influenced by a patient's lifestyle (e.g. when a smoker develops hypertension that, when severe, is a precursor of renal breakdown). Rejection episodes are usually treated in a hospital. If a graft fails completely, the patient has to go through the ordeal of deciding whether to take the risk of another transplant (while usually dialysed at the hospital). Of course, each successive transplantation incurs the renewed possibility of death as well as side-effects or rejection; these risks increase dramatically with the second and each further transplant. As an alternative, a patient can resort to long-term dialysis treatment. But this option carries its own risks while it allows for less normalization of a patient's life than does transplant treatment.

The sociological side of transplantation has been discussed in three different approaches. They focus on the structure of social action from various perspectives, and they emphasize different aspects of the transplantation experience. One is Talcott Parsons', another is symbolic interactionism, and a third is my own work on patient careers in end-stage renal failure.

Parsons's main theme concerning the social context of illness is that health is a functional prerequisite of the system of society (Parsons 1951). In fact, health is the basic guarantor of equality of opportunity in society inasmuch as it makes individuals equal with respect to their capacity to compete with each other in their social roles (Parsons 1958, Gerhardt 1979). This relevance of health for society is mirrored in the sick person's duty to recover, and also in the chronic patient's relentless effort to approximate recovery or avoid deterioration as long as possible (Parsons 1975). In this way, the chronically sick succeed in living a life comparable in many respects to that of normal non-sick members of society.

When writing about kidney transplantation, Parsons stresses two issues. One is that death is involved. It looms large as a prospect that is being shunned or denied while at the same time the transplant, a "gift of life", promises extension and improvement of the patient's existence. The other issue is reciprocity. To be sure, it is the principle of social action as such. In case of transplantation, however, it takes on a particular form that is partly akin to the "gift complex" analyzed by Richard Titmuss and others; Parsons et al. write:

> With the possible exception of "giving birth", and to a lesser extent, donating blood, transplantation entails the most literal "gift of life" that a person can proffer or receive. The donor (a significant linguistic usage) contributes a vital part of his (her) body to a terminally ill, dying recipient, in order to save and maintain that other person's life. Because of the magnitude of this gift-exchange, and its symbolic, as well as biomedical implications, participating in a transplantation can be a transcendent experience for those involved, be it the live donor, the recipient, their relatives, the cadaver donor's family, or the members of the medical team (Parsons et al. 1972/1978: 296).

Symbolic interactionism in contrast addresses the topic of illness using a career perspective. Goffman and early "grounded theory" propose a notion of sickness where a stigma manifests itself in a role that must be taken and draws the person into a spiral of losses (Goffman 1963, Glaser & Strauss 1968). The sick role, from this vantage point, entails a career of progressive deterioration of self (Scheff 1966). Since the 1980s, "grounded theory" has abandoned the idea of career, and it now envisages individuals' sickness as an illness trajectory. The latter is experienced by the patient but it also denotes typical changes characteristic for the course of a particular disease (Corbin & Strauss 1987). The question of self and identity prevails in a recent revision of the approach (Charmaz 1990). The problem is how personal identity can be preserved when practically all social worlds of a patient are jeopardized (Morgan 1988). As Kutner finds, in end-stage renal failure (ESRF) family relationships and friendships as well as job and occupation are affected. In this situation, she states, whether or not a patient can muster the changes depends on family members', employers' etc. "accepting ESRD and its treatment demands" (Kutner 1987: 67).

My own work builds on both approaches. Parsons's ideas are followed when the chronic patient is seen as a person attempting to lead a life that resembles that of normal non-sick members of society as closely as possible. In this vein, social normality becomes equivalent to the normalization that chronic patients accomplish when they participate fully in work and family roles. The notion of socio-economic coping is introduced to highlight patients' efforts to protect and improve their family's socio-economic status-position such that social normality ensues. This means not only that the job and income situation but also family relationships may be rearranged to accommodate for a husband/father's renal failure (Gerhardt 1985, 1986, 1990). The aim is to enable the family to continue to be "normal" despite the main breadwinner's major disease (if at all feasible).

The symbolic interactionist idea of career is reinterpreted. End-stage renal failure, as a major chronic illness, is seen as a *temporal* structure. The latter characterizes the disease process and also the management of the illness. This involves temporal structures on five dimensions of biography; they are: (1) the patient's body, disease and treatment, (2) both spouses's work and occupation, (3) the financial situation of the family, (4) the couple's marriage and friendships, (5) the patient's leisure activities and other areas of self-expression relevant to their personal identity (e.g. holidays, sports). Medical, occupational (including financial) and marital biographies denote *status* biographies.

These status biographies are experienced by the patients as representations of, or deviations from, veritable career patterns. Regarding the three biographies of illness/treatment, work/occupation and marriage, the various statuses experienced in the biographies carry a certain degree of acceptability relative to others. For instance, to be married may be given a higher value than to be divorced, widowed, etc.; to have a job securing high prestige and income may be preferred over a low-level job with reduced prestige and low pay; to have a functioning transplant is preferred over dialysis as treatment status, and among the two modes, a live-donor transplant is "better" than a cadaver-donor transplant. To be sure, this does not mean that patients would not choose a less-than-optimal option under given circumstances. However, they have internalized a "hierarchy" of evaluation of the various biographical status options denoting the latter's presumptive "quality". In the temporal flow of the patient biography, the various options can be experienced for any length of time. What matters is that *careers* are optimal, and patients prefer careers if they can, which means that they attempt to optimize their choices of treatment and other statuses. Careers represent *optimal* patterns of status achievement or status sequence(s). Career-prone biographical constellations are what is deemed successful, and such constellations (which are achieved) represent best options. Biographies contain the orientational perspective of careers. Treatment careers represent what patients strive to reach, and when their treatment biographies deviate from the career pattern, they find important reasons to legitimize why they could not realize the optimal option (Gerhardt 1991a,b).

Empirically, treatment biographies rarely are fully fledged treatment careers. But there are constant changes in biographies that tend toward careers. In my article "Family rehabilitation and longterm survival in end-stage renal failure", I argue that over time a growing number and proportion of surviving patients reach a biographical constellation that is a "survival-optimal" patient career. It consists of a biographical constellation combining a functioning transplant with full-time employment. Measured at an early point in time of the observed patient biography, full-time employment turns out to be a predictor of an increased likelihood of subsequent transplantation that may occur as "late" as ten years after onset of (dialysis) treatment, eventually securing a "survival-optimal" patient career (Gerhardt 1991c).

In the context of patient biographies, the experiences of the patients depend on open-ended coping in a situation of unrelenting uncertainty. Transplants can be received after a relatively limited period of dialysis (usually hospital dialysis), or they may be sought after a more extended period of dialysis including home dialysis. Transplants can be live-donor or cadaver-donor transplants, and they may be successful for only a short time period, or for a long time. When a transplant fails, a next transplant may be available or denied. The treatment option of a live-donor transplant functioning successfully may be desired by most patients, but it is only reached by some. The situation of choice of optimum-option treatment, even when it occurs, is fraught with uncertainty regarding the fate or "success" of the graft. In fact, even a recipient of a long-term successful transplant can never be one hundred per cent sure that rejection of the graft would not happen sooner or later. Moreover, such rejection, if of a live-donor organ, carries the burden of the patient's body's rejecting a "gift of life" received from a family member.

This chapter documents the experience of transplant patients through *interview-narratives*. Tape-recorded data material is used to show how their career orientation works and also how their images of normality are woven into the fabric of discourse accounting for their experiences that make up their biographies. As a focal theme, I concentrate on patients' experience of their option for a transplant, in terms of their narratives on how they came to experience.

Illness-narratives have received sociological attention since the early 1980s. In the British context, Bury (1982) demonstrates how disruption and repair of biographies occur through talk in cases of rheumatoid arthritis (RA), and Williams (1984) shows how "narrative reconstruction" accounting for the genesis of RA serves to re-establish sufferers' sense of self and their integration into their social worlds. In an American context, however, broader issues are stressed. Brody (1987) argues that "stories of sickness" are indispensable when patients or their relatives or doctor(s) make sense of the course and prognosis of their illness. Using partly anthropological material, Kleinman (1988) clarifies that the narrative form of accounting for an illness and its vicissitudes is an intercultural endowment of humankind. From this perspective, narratives reconcile patients' bodies with their biography and also with the culture of which they are part.

If illness-narratives account for the experience of transplant patients under a career perspective, linguistic structures must be found that mirror the optimal-form orientation of the organization of biographical material.

In narrative interviews, as Mishler (1986) points out, respondents account for their experiences and activities by presenting themselves as competent social actors. They picture their biographical particulars under the perspective that they are actors as normal as anybody else – or, on the other hand, exceptional and therefore different from all or most others. The presentation follows a logic of taking-the-role-of-the-other insofar as the narration addresses the *interviewer*. It is the interviewer who should become convinced through the narrative that the narrator (respondent) is a "typical" or, alternatively, an "exceptional" social actor. Life-data are presented in an interview-narrative, Mishler says, such that the interviewer becomes convinced that the respondent as an actor is competent. In this vein, competence of an actor is being constructed by an interviewer on the basis of a narrative presented. Social normality is therefore an interactive accomplishment. For example, in a medical sociological study, Voysey (1972) shows how accounts for a child's disability given by parents (including accounts clad in stories) prove to a family's neighbours etc. but also to an interviewer that the respondents nevertheless are a normal family.

Regarding treatment modes for end-stage renal failure, dialysis and transplantation are the two main forms, but six options are available (live-donor transplant, cadaver-donor transplant, home dialysis, hospital dialysis, continuous ambulatory peritoneal dialysis (CAPD) at home, and CAPD at the hospital). My topic, however, is transplant patients' interview-narratives. How do transplant recipients account for their choice of the best or second-best option? Their accounts include narratives on the option(s) rejected or abandoned as well as on how they came to obtain a transplant. Option(s) abandoned usually include dialysis experience. Practically every transplant patient is dialysed before being transplanted, as the first treatment mode early in his or her biography of end-stage renal failure. A large proportion of patients continue dialysis for extended periods of time subsequent to their onset of treatment before they may be transplanted at a (much) later point in time.

Patients' interview-narratives deal with three relevant themes. They are (1) dialysis experience, (2) family member or physician offering a kidney, (3) transplantation (where the "gift" relationship between donor and recipient may or may not matter). These three themes are dealt with in accounts in the interviews. The latter are here reproduced in text excerpts dealing mainly with the first of the three themes. The interview-narrative, I hypothesize, documents the competence of a social actor who is a transplant patient who "tells his or her story". The result is a construction of a patient's normal personhood in interview material picturing the dialogue between the patient and the interviewer.

The data upon which this chapter is based are drawn from the study *Patient careers in end-stage renal failure* (Gerhardt 1981) (financed by the Social Science Research Council, London, between 1977 and 1980, and the German National Research Council, Bonn, between 1981 and 1982). The study investigated the (near) entire patient population of male, married, 20–50-year-old (at onset) end-stage renal-failure patients who had been treated for not longer than three years at a certain date (1 January 1978) at one of the five teaching hospitals serving the South-East of England. The patients and their wives were interviewed separately twice, one year apart. Interviews were tape-recorded, 234 interviews were conducted that comprise over 600 hours of tape-recorded material.

This chapter uses interview material from the first-wave interviews of four patients who received their first transplants. Their interview-narratives are analyzed using the method of narrative analysis explicated by Mishler (1986).

To make verbatim text easy to use for comparative understanding of meaning structures, text presentation has been introduced by Mishler (1986). He took the method from Chafe (1980). The point is that "meaning units" are identified in the verbatim text transcript, and each "meaning unit" is placed on a separate line of the transcript documentation. This enables the researcher to distinguish relatively easily between the "meaning units", even when they consist only of a single word or a half-finished sentence. The "meaning units" are placed into consecutive lines, which allow for an identification of each "meaning unit" and also of the "meaning episodes" that are made up of several "meaning units". "Meaning episodes", to be sure, frequently are narratives. The method of their representation adapted from Chafe (1980) allows for their identification as *storied narratives*, or as *argumentative narratives*.

The narratives

The following data are taken from the first-wave interviews with two cases who underwent live-donor transplantation (P 09, P 41), and two cases who received a cadaver-donor transplant (P 02, P 47). Two of the cases have in common that they were transplanted after a relatively short period of dialysis in hospital (P 02 and P 09), one had peritoneal dialysis at home for several months (P 41) and one had an extended period of home dialysis before receiving his cadaver-donor transplant (P 47). All cases were interviewed at the beginning of an incumbency of a successful transplant inasmuch as their grafts were to function for a number of years subsequent to their interviews. At the last follow-up, nine years after their first-wave interviews, one of the live-donor kidney recipients (P 41) and one of the cadaver-donor kidney recipients (P 47) were alive with their transplants still working, whereas one live-donor transplant patient (P 09) had died in the previous year after his transplant had functioned for nearly a decade, and one cadaver-donor transplant patient (P 02, a Spaniard) had returned to his home country, apparently after his graft had failed and he expected renewed transplantation in Spain.

Excerpts from the patients' interviews are analyzed here in regard to narratives that relate to their choice of treatment mode. The narratives are presented verbatim in "meaning units" before they are interpreted as "tales of normality".

The live-donor transplant cases had the following characteristics:

CASE No. 9: Received transplant from his older brother.
Age at onset: 37 years; age at transplantation: 37 years.
Family: Married with four children.
Occupation: Lorry driver, unemployed.
Social class: III (non-manual).
CASE No. 41: Received transplant from his sister.
Age at onset: 26 years; age at transplantation: 26 years.
Family: Married with no children.
Occupation: Welder, unemployed.
Social class: III (manual).

CASE No. 9 narrative

[1] I: So you were not dialysed

[2] when you were in (Local Hospital)

[3] P: no

[4] I was just on the P. B.

[5] P. B. is it

[6] I: oh yes peritoneal

[7] P: yea

[8] the bottles

[9] yea

[10] they push in your stomach

[11] you know

[12] they done that

[13] when I was in the (Local Hospital)

[14] I: yes

[15] but that is a kind of dialysis

[16] P: yea yea

[17] it's like

[18] I: and so they transferred you to (Metropolitan Hospital)

[19] P: yes

[20] when they had

[21] yea

[22] when they had room like

[23] transferred me over to East Suburb

[24] then they put me on the bags again

[25] over there

[26] oh I think for about two or three weeks

[27] then they put the shunt in me leg

[28] and then

[29] as I say

[30] I was on the machine twice a week

[31] I was only on for six hours a time

[32] I: which is quite a short time

[33] P: yea

[34] 'cause everybody else was nine hours

[35] three times a week

[36] as I say

[37] I was only on twice

[38] I: do you know why

[39] P: no

[40] so fit

[41] that's what he used to tell me

[42] I used to walk up the ward

147

[43] with me
[44] you know
[45] the bags
[46] I used to push me trolley
[47] up the ward with them
[48]I: oh that's incredible
[49]P: yes
[50] well he said that
[51] Dr Waller
[52] used to say
[53] you're incredible
[54] if I went to go to the toilet
[55] I would just get out of bed
[56] and push me trolley with me bags
[57] and take it with me
[58]I: fantastic
[59] so you're very fit
[60] and you really
[61]P: yea
[62] they said
[63] they'd never seen a patient like me
[64] I don't know why
[65] I don't know
[66] if I'm bionic
[67]I: you know some people
[68] they're very weak
[69] they are very very weak
[70] they can't walk stairs
[71]P: he said to me
[72] you know
[73] you're fantastic
[74]I: oh that's great
[75] and so you came home
[76] after five weeks in hospital
[77]P: yea
[78] something like that
[79] then I had to go back
[80] like twice a week
[81] the ambulance used to pick me up
[82] from the machine
[83] then
[84] I don't suppose
[85] I was on the machine for

[86] eight or nine times
[87]I: do you exactly remember
[88] how often you were
[89] when you actually went over
[90] from [Local Hospital] to [Metropolitan Hospital]
[91] when that was
[92] can you exactly remember the dates
[93] or just about what month it was
[94]P: January
[95]I: January (this year)
[96] this year yea
[97] about 18th
[98] I think
[99] or 19th
[100] I think it was 19th
[101] 'cause everything happened on the 19th
[102] 19th January
[103] then I had me transplant
[104] on March 19th
[105] so say
[106] it was two months
[107] I was messed about like.
(P 9 I, A 82–142).

The action story line of the narrative about P 9's dialysis experience leading up to his transplantation shows three stages of treatment that form a succession ranging from undesirable option to best option. The peritoneal dialysis that is not even acknowledged as dialysis is followed by haemodialysis that is followed by the transplant. The three stages in the treatment biography culminating in the transplant operation are: P. D. at the local hospital (lines 1–17), transfer to East Suburb hospital that is part of Metropolitan Hospital where the transplant operation took place, where the patient was treated by haemodialysis (18–86), and eventually transplantation as the peak and culminating point of it all (87–104). As a resolution, he sums up his dialysis experience as having lasted only two months and nevertheless having been utterly undesirable, by saying "I was messed about like" (107).

Interspersed into the story line of successful attainment of a live-donor transplant are evaluations. Each of the three complications, to use the Labov–Waletzki (1967) frame of narrative analysis, carries an evaluation that connects the story line with its culmination point, the transplant. The first complication (P. D. in local hospital) carries the evaluation of not having been right for this patient that he expresses by diminishing it to not even being dialysis ("I was just on P. B.", 4; incidentally, he persistently misspells the treatment acronym). The second complication (haemodialysis at East Suburb Hospital) carries the evaluation of P's being exceptionally fit. He proves by his favourable treatment schedule that he must have been fitter than the ordinary dialysis patient. He thus implies that he must have been fitter than is required if a patient can expect nothing but dialysis. His fitness is exemplified by two narrative proofs, namely, his physical independence that everybody could observe ("push me trolley up the ward", 46/7, 56), and the staff's laudatory comments about his fitness. To prove that the latter were no empty flatter he invokes his own amazement about the degree of his fitness by the evaluation "I don't know if I'm bionic" (66). The third complication (live-donor transplantation at Metropolitan Hospital) needs no justification; it "speaks for itself", so to speak; he simply draws a slightly magic connection between the dates of his referral and of his operation.

CASE No. 41 narrative:
1 I: So Dr Goldberg said
2 that it was possible for you
3 to go on a machine
4 P: yea
5 I: and that was
6 P: give give me hope
7 I had to wait for me turn
8 you know
9 wait for the machine which
10 I went on P. D.
11 I: this was in what
12 October
13 P: uhm
14 soon as I was in hospital
15 about two days after
16 I was on P. D.
17 which was terrible
18 you know
19 I: was it
20 P: yea
21 you know
22 the pipe in the stomach
23 it was
24 I was in the bed
25 four days a week you know
26 and had the weekend at home
27 and when I come home
28 I had to just sit all the time

[29] couldn't go out
[30] 'cause the pipe was still in there like
[31]I: did it bother you
[32] the pipe
[33] was it sort of painful
[34]P: well it was painful yea
[35] you was frightened to sleep
[36] most of the time
[37] 'cause you might roll over on it
[38] and push it in too far
[39] and things like that
[40]I: could people see it
[41] like when you walked down the street
[42] people would
[43]P: well I used to have an elastic band
[44] over the top of my trousers
[45] with the zip half way down
[46] so the pipe was sticking out
[47] and I used to have a big jumper
[48] over the top
[49] so I didn't really pull against it
[50] and it was really terrible
[51] you know
[52] if I went shopping with me wife
[53] I used to have to walk behind
[54] all the time
[55] 'cause I was frightened
[56] of people walking into me
[57] you know
[58] but I was on that
[59] for six months
[60]I: so that
[61] all the time
[62] you were four days a week
[63] in the hospital
[64]P: actually I was on P. D.
[65] Monday and Tuesday
[66] I had a day off
[67] you know
[68] off the bed
[69] I could go and sit in the day room
[70] then I was on
[71] Thursday and Friday

[72] then I had Saturday and Sunday at home
[73] you know
[74] really terrible
[75] but it was better than nothing
[76] you know
[77] keeping me alive
[78] that was the main thing
(P 41 I, A 60–1)

The patient here tells the story of his P. D.; elsewhere in his interview he tells a similarly dismal story of his subsequent haemodialysis. Both narratives document that the patient is not suitable for dialysis treatment. The logical conclusion, to be sure, is that the only adequate treatment mode for him is a transplant – and a live-donor transplant even, which is the best possible option. His narrative concerning his terrible experience of P. D. is immediately followed in the interview text by the sentence: "Six months later they put me on the machine but in that time me sister offered me a kidney" (P 41 I, A 1–102).

As for the lack of suitability of this patient for dialysis – here P. D. –, the action story line is to give *negative* proof. The narrative starts with an overall evaluation (1–18) summing up the treatment's value as just giving him hope (6), which corresponds to the narrative's resolution that the treatment is only worthy because it kept him alive (77–8). The narrative unfolds through three episodes that are reactions to the interviewer's probing. First, P responds to the interviewer's probe why P. D. was terrible. He clarifies that he had to be in his hospital bed most of the time, and at home he could only sit (that is, he stresses his loss of capacity to stand or walk). Then, he responds to the question whether P. D. was painful; he clarifies that it was frightening (that is, he points at his loss of capacity to do normal things such as sleep). Thirdly, he responds to the question whether his disability was publicly visible; he recalls how he went out partly undressed and how he hid behind his wife when they went shopping (that is, he mentions his loss of capacity to be a partner for his wife). The interviewer, having understood now that the three answers corroborate the evidence of his non-suitability for P. D., accepts P's negative evaluation. She signals that she no longer questions his judgement, by returning to the matter of her first question that reacted to P's characterization of P. D. as "terrible" (60ff.). He responds by closing the narrative, reiterating how unacceptable the time schedule was, which also was his first proof of lack of suitability of P. D. for him (see above). He then states again his evaluation that the treatment was terrible, and then he closes the entire episode by the story resolution ("keeping me alive that was the main thing").

P 9 talks about his dialysis experience to document that his physical fitness exceeded that of a normal dialysis patient; this suggests that he is suitable for a better treatment than dialysis (indeed, suitable for the best treatment altogether). In contrast, P 41 talks about his dialysis experience to document how the treatment deprived him of the most essential capacities of a person in general and a man and husband in particular. However, both accounts have the function of convincing the interviewer that the patient was suitable for the best-option treatment that he received. The justification of his suitability is either that he was physically exceedingly fit to the extent that he might have appeared "bionic", or that he became physically so unfit that even the normal functions of an adult and a man could no longer be performed. Both narratives, to be sure, affirm that the live-donor transplant treatment for the particular patient was right. P 9 argues that he appeared supra-normal while he was on dialysis but is now normal with a live-donor transplant. P 41 argues that he became subnormal while on dialysis but has recovered to normality subsequent to receiving a live-donor transplant.

In contrast to the live-donor transplant cases, the cadaver-donor transplant cases follow a slightly different logic in order to justify their treatment option. On the one hand, they also have to prove that they are unsuitable for dialysis. On the other hand, however, they have to prove that a live-donor transplant for them is not a viable option. From this double proof given in their narratives, it follows that they have obtained the treatment that is best for them to allow for their leading normal lives.

The *cadaver-donor transplant* cases analyzed here have the following characteristics:

CASE No. 2: CDT after P. D. and haemodialysis at the hospital.
Age at onset: 25 years; age at transplantation: 26 years.
Family: Married with two children.
Occupation: Foreman in a local medium-size firm.
Social class: III (manual).
CASE No. 47: CDT after extended period of home dialysis, with wife as dialysis helper.
Age at onset: 36 years; age at transplantation: 38 years.
Family: Married with two children.
Occupation: Taxi driver.
Social class: III (non-manual).
CASE No. 2 narrative:
[1]I: when did you decide
[2] to go on the transplant list
[3]P: a few months
[4] after they took me into St. Theodore's
[5]I: how did it happen
[6]P: I didn't like the dialysis machine
[7] maybe it was

[8] because they were taking
[9] so much off me
[10] see
[11] and I felt so bad
[12] after
[13] and before
[14] sometimes I used to go
[15] before the time
[16] to hospital
[17] because I couldn't take any more
[18] you know
[19] I was drinking too much
[20] my own fault
[21] and I thought
[22] that it was better
[23] either to have the transplant
[24] or die
[25] before being on the machine
[26] if I have to be on the machine
[27] I think
[28] I prefer to die
[29] if they say to me
[30] you got to be on the machine
[31] all your life
[32] then I'd rather die
[33] than be on the machine
[34] if it's only
[35] you know
[36] my kidneys stop
[37] and say
[38] we get you another one
[39] nice people
[40]I: did you ask
[41] to be put on the transplant list
[42] or did somebody come
[43] and offer it to you
[44] did somebody come round
[45] and say
[46] we could put you on the transplant list
[47] or did you yourself say
[48] listen Dr Hickson
[49] or whoever it was
[50] I want to have a transplant

[51]P: we had to ask Dr Grand
[52] we had to go and see him
[53] and
[54] well
[55] put our name down
[56] for the
[57] put my name down
[58] for the transplant
[59]I: I mean
[60] I guess
[61] you had
[62] for when
[63] and then you
[64]P: and then I decided
[65] I'd do it
[66] transplantation
[67]I: and what did he say
[68] Dr Grand
[69]P: I was in risk of being
[70] you know
[71] I was dying
[72] or something
[73] because I was putting on
[74] so much weight
[75] they used to tell me
[76] every now and again
[77] to drink less
[78] and these things
[79] but I couldn't help it
[80] so they were very glad
[81] that I decided
[82] to do the transplant
[83] they didn't tell me
[84] they wanted me to go
[85] and ask them
[86] they don't want to tell
[87] I don't think
[88] they [don't] want tell anybody
[89] to have a transplant done
[90] but they are glad
[91] that people go to them
[92] and say
[93] I would like to have a transplant

[94] in other words
[95] they want the people
[96] to decide for themselves
[97] see
[98] not the people say
[99] I want a transplant
[100] because you say so
[101] they want
[102] the patient to decide
[103] and I decided
[104] and thank God I did
[105] I: did you at any point
[106] consider asking a relative
[107] for a kidney
[108] or did you always think
[109] you didn't want a relative
[110] you wanted it
[111] from somebody
[112] the hospital knows about
[113] P: well my mother
[114] she was willing
[115] to give me a kidney
[116] but I didn't want it
[117] because
[118] well
[119] if she gives me a kidney
[120] that's to say
[121] if the kidney
[122] doesn't work on me
[123] then I will still be disabled
[124] and probably
[125] my mother starts feeling bad
[126] you know
[127] so I say no
[128] leave it
[129] you keep your own kidneys
[130] and if they give me one
[131] good enough
[132] if not
[133] that's it
(P 2 I, A 11–18)

The action story line in case No. 2 spans from P's negative dialysis experience through his rejection of his mother's offer to donate him a live-donor organ to his active role in carrying out his decision to obtain a cadaver-donor transplant. He uses an argumentative narrative to justify his rejection of dialysis treatment as not suitable for him. The narrative answers to the question how it happened that he went on the hospital's transplant list (which contains the names of the patients waiting for a suitable cadaver-donor kidney to "come up"). He gives two reasons why he is not suitable for dialysis. One is his risk of death brought about by his own inability to adhere to the fluid-reduction regimen imperative for long-term survival on the treatment (14–20); this meant that his weight gain between dialysis sessions was excessive (14–18). This, in turn, meant that he had to be dialysed at a high fluid-extraction rate (8–9) that usually makes patients vomit during and after dialysis sessions (11–13). Second, he justifies his unsuitability for dialysis by his preference for death if he is given no other alternative except dialysis. The option is clearly, "either to have a transplant or die" (23–4); dialysis is not acceptable for him, he reiterates: "I'd rather die than be on the machine" (32–3).

The second step in his action story is his decision not to accept his mother's offer of a live-donor organ (15–133). He again tells an argumentative narrative rather than a full-fledged story, stating the fact(s) and then giving the reason(s). The facts were: "My mother was willing to give me a kidney but I didn't want it" (113–16). The reason is: If this live-donor transplant would fail, the situation would be worse than now, that is, he would be still "disabled" (123), and she could "start feeling bad" (125). From this it follows that he rejected the offer, saying to her (in his narrative): "No, leave it, you keep your own kidneys" (127–9). It is not clear whether the reason he gives for this in the text is what he said to his mother or how he justifies himself vis-à-vis the interviewer: He repeats that his alternatives are cadaver-donor transplantation or death (130–33).

Thirdly, he tells the story of entering his name on the transplant list. It focuses on his own decision and action, showing also that he did what the hospital staff expected him to do. He decided for himself, but this was what the hospital staff usually expected. The story narrative (69–104) consists of four complications, namely, (1) he was in danger of dying due to his failure to control his fluid intake (69–74), (2) he was told to comply but could not (75–9), (3) the staff were glad about his decision (80–82) – that is also an evaluation following from the two previous complications, as may be learned from the "so" at the beginning of line 80 – and (4) the staff usually act in this way (83–93). This leads to the overall evaluation that he acted as he should when he made the decision himself (94–102), followed by the resolution ("and I decided", 103), plus a coda ("and thank God I did", 104).

Preceded by his argumentative statement against dialysis, and preceded by his report on how he rejected his mother's offer, his story narrative justifies his transplant decision for a cadaver-donor organ. The text episode on dialysis suggests that his viable alternatives are transplantation or death. The text episode on the mother's offer and his not accepting it clarifies that the transplant is to be a cadaver-donor one, and the text episode on going on the transplant list confirms how he himself made the decision that was right. He thus pictures himself as a man who has been able to maintain his independence (as a body who avoids dependence on a machine, as a man who decides for himself), and he thereby reassures the interviewer that he has chosen a treatment that gives him normality (as a body, as a man).

CASE No. 47 narrative:

1 I: So was it a choice
2 did you decide
3 to have home dialysis
4 P: oh yes
5 well they give us three choices
6 you know
7 he says to me
8 one you can
9 well
10 two you can have
11 the transplant or the machine
12 he says
13 but I'll give you three choices
14 there's you know
15 one
16 he says
17 we haven't lost anybody on the machine
18 and
19 no
20 how was it he put it
21 I can't remember now
22 yes
23 one
24 he says
25 you can have a transplant
26 two
27 it takes
28 three
29 you die
30 you know what I mean
31 these are the three alternatives
32 you know

[33] well
[34] I says
[35] I don't fancy
[36] the one it doesn't take
[37] I don't fancy
[38] the one you die
[39] so
[40] I says
[41] I'll have the machine
[42] you know
[43] so I accepted it right away
[44] you know
[45] so I says to my wife
[46] I says
[47] we'll have to go on the machine
[48] and we'll give it
[49] you know
[50] four or five years
[51] you know
[52] on the machine
[53] and then
[54] in that time
[55] it can improve
[56] you know
[57] transplant
[58] it can improve
[59] but after a couple of years
[60] my wife was deteriorating
[61] more than I was
[62] you know
[63] I could see the difference in her
[64] you know
[65] because it was a long day for her
[66]I: when you say
[67] she was deteriorating
[68]P: well the point is
[69] you know
[70] she was getting up
[71] in the morning
[72] very early in the morning
[73] and taking
[74] helping to get me off the machine
[75] getting the children ready for school

76 and then going off to work
77 and working very hard
78 at her job
79 coming in in the evening
80 you know
81 feeling very very tired
82 so
83 over a period of over two years
84 you know what I mean
85 she sort of started
86 I could see the difference
87 and that
88 she weren't as fresh and bright
89 as she normally is
90 and that
91 you know
92 and this is
93 when I thought to myself
94 I thought
95 I say to myself
96 well I feel alright
97 you know
98 I feel good
99 and the point is
100 I says to her
101 I says
102 what do you think
103 shall we have a go
104 for a transplant
105 you know
106 so she says
107 well
108 we'll have a chat to them
109 about it
110 and this was the thing
111 but since
112 I've come off the machine
113 and that
114 you know
115 she's starting
116 to feel a lot better now
117 you know what I mean
118I: oh

[119] that's marvellous
[120]P: well
[121] it was more for her
[122] than for myself
[123] you know
[124] that we decided
[125] on having a transplant
(P 47 I: A 66–125).

The action story line in case No. 47 spans from P being given a choice, and choosing home dialysis because it carried the least risks, to eventually abandoning home dialysis in favour of a transplant because his wife (and dialysis helper) suffered more from his home dialysis than he did himself.

The narrative consists of four episodes. The first episode, recollecting his choice between the treatment modes, is a full-fledged story (1–44); he tells how he consciously chose home dialysis. The second episode is argumentative, justifying his suggestion to his wife that they "have the machine"; he argues that it was not unreasonable to think that within four or five years survival chances would have been improved further through medical progress (45–58). The third episode (interrupted and also spurred by the interviewer's probe) again has a story structure; it is abstracted by the statement that the wife was deteriorating more than himself, and when the interviewer wishes to understand what he means, he tells a story. Its first complication represents her mornings and evenings (68–81); its second complication (which follows from the first, as is shown by P starting line 82 by "so") explains her deterioration (83–9). The third represents his reaction to the situation ("I feel good") that, however, is immediately neutralized by a fourth complication that pictures him asking his wife and heeding her advice (90–109). The subsequent evaluation is also the central theme of the narrative, accounting for his having a transplant. He states, as some kind of resolution for the entire narrative, "this was the thing", which means that he was fully right in how he acted and that he had had a transplant (110). The remainder of the narrative is an argumentative evaluation that stresses that he was right by presenting evidence for his decision having been beneficial: his wife feels better. The conclusion emphasizes another aspect that pertains to his normality, namely, that he is a good husband and family man: "it was more for her than for myself that we decided on having the transplant" (121–5).

In both cases of cadaver-donor transplant, to be sure, their treatment is second-best among the "hierarchy" of options (although neither of them seems to have been keen on a live-donor transplant). P 2 justifies his not being on dialysis by his extremely negative experience with the treatment, and his not having a live-donor transplant by actively having rejected an offer. P 47, in fact, opted for dialysis that he found a thoroughly positive experience; only when his wife and dialysis helper began to "deteriorate" due to *her* negative experience with his treatment did P decide actively to seek a transplant. Whereas P 2 argues that the transplant was right for him because otherwise he would have died, P 47 argues that *he* was right when he realized that it was to his wife's benefit if and when he was transplanted. As a person and husband, he put his wife's suffering over his own wellbeing.

Both patients report that they made their deliberate choices themselves. It was they who independently came to the conclusion that it was indispensable (P 2) or wise (P 47) to seek transplantation. P 2 is convinced that to be a person requires the normality that only a transplant can offer. P 47 is convinced that to continue to be the husband and father that he is means that the risk had to be taken to voluntarily expose himself to a transplant operation. In case 2, the patient knew that to survive required transplantation, in case P 47 this was not so. P 47 *could* have continued on home dialysis; but it would have meant him losing the family life that he loves and seeing his wife deteriorate still further as a consequence of his not being able or willing to change his treatment type.

Discussion: the social issue of normality

The "gift of life", whether received from a relative as live-donor transplant or from an anonymous stranger as a cadaver-donor transplant, is not a normal event. However, it is the best attainable way for a person with end-stage renal failure to preserve or resume normality as a social actor. In this respect, transplantation is superior to any other treatment of end-stage renal failure.

Following Parsons's idea that the "gift of life" involves a relationship of reciprocity, we may return to the question of what that reciprocation consists of. My hypothesis is that the patient who receives a "gift of life" that is known to allow for a return to a relatively perfect normal life (or a relatively normal life, for that matter) feels responsible for accomplishing as much normality as he or she can muster. That is, the patient's part in the reciprocity relationship between kidney donor and recipient consists of "being worthy". If he or she is to "deserve" the gift received, so to speak, he or she is obliged to prove it by accomplishing as much of a return to normality as he or she can manage.

To be sure, the "gift" relationship is not necessarily of a personal nature. Not only do cadaver-donor graft recipients not know who "gave them life" (the principle of anonymity of donorship being strictly observed by the hospital staff), but live-donor kidney recipients who do know who their donor was do not express in their interviews that they are particularly grateful to their relatives who helped them to live through an organ donation. Rather, they are grateful to the physician who appears to them more important for their transplantation than their organ donors. Accordingly, live-donor graft recipients seem to feel and act in a strikingly similar way to recipients of cadaver-donor grafts whose donors remain anonymous. This suggests that there is a similarity of the *social* relationship between donor and recipient, irrespective of whether or not there exists a personal or blood relationship. This social relationship, epitomized in the formula of the "gift of life", suggests that a *societal* duty is felt by a person who has received an organ transplant.

This societal duty, I assume, is that these patients experience responsibility for "being worth it". That a patient understands this responsibility is documented through their expressing in the interview that they achieved what they were supposed to achieve – i.e. normality. The graft recipient's successfully returning to utmost possible normality is their social duty following recipiency of an organ transplant. In this vein, normality as a person and/or as a man is the proof within the "gift relationship" that a recipient has been "worth" the "gift of life" received. It is society as "conscience collective", to adopt Durkheim's perspective, which here is the agency or addressee whose expectations are thus being met.

In our interview material, the patients have to show on two counts that they understand their responsibility of "being worth it". Their return to utmost feasible normality is argued in their interviews with respect to two related but separate issues. One is that they know about the "hierarchy" of treatment modes that puts live-donor transplantation above cadaver-donor transplantation, and both above any kind of dialysis. The other is that they must prove how normal they have become (or have always been) through convincing the interviewer that they *are* normal men.

With regard to "being worth" the top-type treatment, a live-donor graft recipient must prove in his interview that he is "worth" the best possible renal replacement therapy – and maybe he is more worthy of it than if he were just a cadaver-donor recipient. Patient 9 accomplishes this by dramatically emphasizing his physical fitness; for him it is sufficient justification for only the highest-order treatment type that he is physically so fit that one might come to think that he is somebody "out of this world" – he refers to himself as some kind of "bionic man". Patient 41 accomplishes it by another strategy of overdramatization. He draws a drastic picture of his suffering when on dialysis that puts into focus the serendipitous improvement brought about by the transplant received from his sister. He claims to have "moved up" from baby-like incapacity (being unable to stand or walk), pathology-like disability (being too frightened to even go to sleep), and child-like unmanliness ("trailing" his wife in public).

Cadaver-donor recipients, by contrast, cannot necessarily prove how normal they are by simply justifying their mode of transplant treatment. Because cadaver-donor transplantation is only the "second-best" option, these patients must prove separately that their treatment is right for *them*, and that they have returned to, or indeed never lost, their social normality as a man. Patient 2 gives an argumentative account of how he rejected his mother's offer to donate an organ. He argues that he was the one who declined on the offer, out of responsibility for the future relationship with his mother considering that her donated organ could "not work on him". Having thus given a plausible reason for why he has not received top-type treatment (whereby he is vindicated as a rational man), he proceeds to account for his rejection of the lesser options of treatment (dialysis of any kind) by dramatically picturing how he always preferred death over dialysis.

Patient 47 does not mention live-donor transplantation at all. Maybe he feels that he would not be expected to justify why he had no first-choice treatment but why he has had the transplantation since he did not "need" it: he was not in danger of dying (or wishing to die, for that matter) nor in dismal physical or psychological shape when he finished his two-year dialysis treatment. In fact, he "felt good" on the machine. So it would not be rational to pretend now that he opted out of his home dialysis and "moved up" to transplant treatment due to his incapacity or other physical or psychological handicaps. He invokes his normality because he needs to justify having taken a risk when he opted for a transplant. His normality thus invoked is social, not physical; it is his identity as a husband and father that is being preserved and reinforced by his voluntary change from dialysis to transplantation.

All four cases give narrative proof of their normality. They take into account what the treatment option is and relate it to these patients' bodily and social identities, using argumentative as well as storied narratives in the interviews. These patients thus manage to document to the interviewer (who is a woman) that they have fulfilled their social obligation upon receiving a "gift of life" – they have returned to or never ceased being a normal man.

References

Brody, H. 1987. *Stories of sickness*. New Haven and London: Yale University Press.

Bury, M. 1982. Chronic illness as biographical disruption. *Sociology of Health and Illness* 4, 167–82.

Chafe, W. L. 1980. *The Pear stories. Cognitive, cultural, and linguistic aspects of narrative production.* Norwood, NJ: Ablex.

Challand, C. 1972. Iatrogenic problems of end-stage renal failure. *New England Journal of Medicine* **287**, 334–6.

Charmaz, K. 1990. "Discovering" chronic illness: using grounded theory. *Social Science and Medicine* **3**, 1161–72.

Corbin, J. & A. Strauss 1987. Accompaniment of chronic illness: changes in body, self, biography, and biographical time. In *Research in the sociology of health care*, vol. 6: *The experience and management of chronic illness*, J. Roth & P. Conrad (eds), 249–91. Greenwich, Connecticut. JAI Press.

Fox, R. & J. Swazey 1974. *The courage to fail: a survival view of organ transplants and dialysis.* Chicago: University of Chicago Press.

Gerhardt, U. 1979. The Parsonian paradigm and the identity of medical sociology. *Sociological Review* (New Series) **22**, 229–51.

Gerhardt, U. 1981. *Patient careers in end-stage renal failure.* End of Grant report No 513. London: Social Science Research Council.

Gerhardt, U. 1985. Family rehabilitation in end-stage renal failure. In *Proceedings of the European Dialysis and Transplant Nurses Association, 13th Congress held in Florence, Italy, 1984*, E. Stevens & P. Monkhouse (eds), 87–95. London: Pitman Medical.

Gerhardt, U. 1986. *Patientenkarrieren. Eine medizinsoziologische Studie.* Frankfurt: Suhrkamp.

Gerhardt, U. 1990. Patient careers in end-stage renal failure. *Social Science and Medicine* **3**, 1211–24.

Gerhardt, U. 1991a. Idealtypische Analyse von Statusbiographien bei chronisch Kranken. In *Gesellschaft und Gesundheit*, 9–6. Frankfurt: Suhrkamp.

Gerhardt, U. 1991b. Chronische Erkrankung: Handlungsrationalität und das Problem der sozialen Pathologie. In *Gesellschaft und Gesundheit*, 61–87. Frankfurt: Suhrkamp.

Gerhardt, U. 1991c. Family rehabilitation and longterm survival in end-stage renal failure. In *Advances in medical sociology*, vol. 2, G. Albrecht & J. Levy (eds), 25–244. Greenwich, Connecticut: JAI Press.

Glaser, B. & A. Strauss 1968. *Time for dying.* Chicago: Aldine.

Goffman, E. 1963. *Stigma. Notes on the management of spoiled identity.* New York: Doubleday.

Kleinman, A. 1988. *The illness narratives. Suffering, healing, and the human condition.* New York: Basic Books.

Kutner, N. G. 1987. Social worlds and identity in end-stage renal disease ESRD. In *Research in the sociology of health care*, vol. 6: *The experience and management of chronic illness*, J. Roth & P. Conrad (eds), 33–72. Greenwich, Connecticut: JAI Press.

Labov, W. & J. Waletzki 1967. Narrative analysis: oral versions of personal experience. In *Essays on the verbal and visual arts. Proceedings of the 1966 annual spring meeting of the American Ethnological Society*, J. Helm (ed.), 12–44. Seattle: University of Washington.

Mishler, E. 1986. The analysis of interview-narratives. In *Narrative psychology. The storied nature of human conduct*, T. R. Sarbin (ed.), 233–55. New York: Praeger.

Morgan, J. 1988. Living with renal failure on home hemodialysis. In *Living with chronic illness. The experience of patients and their families*, R. Anderson & M. Bury (eds), 23–224. London: Unwin Hyman.

Parsons, T. 1951. *The social system*. Glencoe, Illinois: Free Press.

Parsons, T. 1958. The definition of health and illness in the light of American values and social structure. In *Patients, physicians and illness*, E. Gartly Jaco (ed.), 122–44. Chicago: University of Chicago Press.

Parsons, T. 1975. The sick role and the role of the physician reconsidered. *Milbank Memorial Fund Quarterly* **53**, 257–78.

Parsons, T., R. Fox, V. Lidz 1972. The "gift of life" and its reciprocation. *Social Research* **39**, 367–415. Reprinted in: Parsons, T. 1978. *Action theory and the human condition*, 264–99. New York: Free Press.

Scheff, T. 1966. *Being mentally ill: a sociological theory*. Chicago: Aldine.

Simmons, R., S. D. Klein, R. L. Simmons 1977. *Gift of life: the social and psychological impact of organ transplantation*. New York: Wiley.

Voysey, M. 1972. *A constant burden. The reconstitution of family life*. London: Routledge & Kegan Paul.

Williams, G. 1984. The genesis of chronic illness: narrative reconstruction. *Sociology of Health and Illness* **6**, 175–200.

Chapter 8
A "failure" of modern medicine?
Lay perspectives on a pain relief clinic

Gillian A. Bendelow

A primary role of medicine is often perceived to be the treatment or alleviation of pain, but what actually constitutes pain is open to a multitude of definitions and interpretation. Pain relief in medical practice tends to concentrate on the nociceptive or sensory aspects of pain, employing the acute/chronic differentiation, and is often unable to encompass the more social and emotional aspects of chronic pain. It is universally acknowledged that one of the most complex and difficult types of pain to treat is "idiopathic" pain, that is, "pain in which there is no sign of tissue damage and for which there is no agreed cause (such as most low back pains and headaches including migraine)" (Melzack & Wall 1988: 165). Kotarba (1983) has charted the process of adjustment to chronic pain and becoming a "pain-afflicted" person in order to trace the continuity of personal identity. Using pain biographies he identified three stages in this process. First, there is the "onset" stage, which is perceived to be transitory, and able to be dealt with by diagnosis and treatment. Here, pain is diagnosed as "real" by physicians, having a physiological basis. The second stage concerns what Kotarba terms the "emergence of doubt". At this stage, treatment may not work, there is an increase in specialist consultations, but patients still feel in control in seeking the best care available. Finally, the third stage concerns what Kotarba terms the "chronic pain experience". Following the shortcomings of treatment, the patient, at this stage, may return to the lay frame of reference, and seek help within the "chronic pain sub-culture" (Kotarba 1983: 27). This experience, often termed *chronic pain syndrome*, and the elusive search for cure or relief may dominate a person's life and inevitably results in a long-term process of the medicalization of their predicament.

This chapter is concerned with the treatment of chronic pain, often described as one of the most difficult and frustrating of medical problems, but concentrates on the views of those experiencing the treatment as opposed to those administering it. In doing so, it aims to switch the focus from supposedly "objective" clinical perspectives to more subjective "lay" accounts and experiences of treatment. As such, it is rooted in an interpretive sociological perspective concerning the meaning and *experience* of chronic illness in which concepts such as "biographical disruption" (Bury 1982), "narrative reconstruction" (Williams 1984) and "styles of adjustment" (Herzlich 1973, Radley & Green 1987) come to the fore (Bury 1991). This focus on the person, rather than measuring so-called objective symptoms, allows us more readily to encompass the notion of *total* pain (Saunders 1976), which includes psychological, spiritual, interpersonal and even financial, as well as physical aspects, of chronic pain.

Increasingly, lay beliefs about pain are acknowledged to have an important effect on patient "satisfaction" and "compliance" with medical care and therapeutic interventions (Williams & Thorn 1989). Consequently, there has been a shift towards more "biographical" forms of medicine that emphasize patient subjectivity and locate pain in a psychosocial context (Armstrong 1983, Arney & Neill 1983, Nettleton 1992). It is in this context that multidisciplinary pain clinics have evolved bringing mind and body into a new alliance. However, as we shall see below, despite such developments, it remains debatable how much the attempt to transcend the mind/body dualism extends to actual treatment and therapy.

Pain clinics or pain centres are institutions that have been developed specifically for the treatment of chronic pain conditions. As Sarafino (1991) emphasizes, before the 1970s, if people's pain lingered and their physician could not determine its cause or find a remedy for the discomfort, these patients were left with virtually no reasonable treatment alternatives. In desperation, the finding of extreme solutions was not infrequent, leading to drug addiction, or irreversible nerve damage. In this respect, Sarafino implies that the evolution and development of pain clinics has given rise to effective alternatives.

The concept of having special institutions for treating pain originated with John Bonica, an anaesthetist in the USA, who recommended in *The management of pain* (1953) that the treatment and understanding of pain would be best achieved through the co-operation of different disciplines. The first pain clinic was set up in the USA in 1961 with specialists from 13 different disciplines, aiming to collaborate in a non-hierarchical manner. The subsequent developments of pain centres throughout North America and Europe vary, not only in terms of provision and resources, but also concerning the organization of work, medical specialities, working principles and therapies. They can be private organizations, or affiliated to medical schools, university departments or hospitals, and may incorporate a variety of treatment methods, or adopt just one approach. Indeed, a cross-sectional survey of 25 pain centres in a single urban community in the USA (Csordas & Clark 1992) found that there were wide variations in the treatment modalities offered, the types of pain conditions treated, the populations served, the patient selections criteria and the diagnostic and aetiologic frames of reference. The study also examined pain centres and clinics across the whole of the USA and identified three different types. First, they found multidisciplinary, comprehensive pain centres, which are dedicated to all kinds of pain problems and offer a wide range of treatment modalities. Secondly, there were syndrome-orientated centres, which only treat one particular kind of pain problem (e.g. headache or back pain). Finally, there were modality-orientated treatment centres that offered only one type of treatment modality, such as analgesic nerve blocks (Csordas & Clark 1992: 385).

In contrast to these American studies, research in the European context on the treatment of pain in clinics has been rare. A notable exception here concerns a study in the Netherlands by Vrancken (1989). Vrancken examined the theory and practice of pain in eight academic pain centres, and identified *five* broad approaches to both theoretical and practical aspects of pain. First, there is the *somatico-technical* approach, adopting a neurophysiological model. Here, pain is viewed as organic, with great emphasis on its classification. Within this approach, time is the only distinction made between acute and chronic pain. Treatment consists mainly of surgical procedures to eradicate, block or ease pain. Consequently, the long-term use of narcotics and the development of secondary psychological complications are seen as second rate. Within this treatment modality, patients are cured when objective signs disappear. Secondly, the *dualistic body-orientated* approach sees pain as a result of organic, psychological and social factors. In this model, there is supposedly no distinction between the body and the mind in theory. However, in practice, although other factors are seen to affect the final expression of pain, the nociceptive (i.e. the purely sensory) aspect is the major factor and methodological dualism tends to be reflected in the physical forms of treatment offered. Again, the patient is cured when the pain is gone. The *behaviourist* approach is used by psychologists where pain is seen to be chronic and intractable, consisting of overt actions that constitute "pain behaviour", as distinct from acute nociceptive pain treated by physicians. In other words, the pain is "in the mind", with all the negative implications of being "imaginary" and the patient is deemed to have recovered when the pain behaviour is replaced by effective "well behaviour".

The remaining two approaches move even further away from scientific medicine. The *phenomenological* approach sees pain as a complex of reactions and behaviours, triggered as a physiological self-defence under harmful conditions, but in its course independent of the initial event – the "pain function". Chronic pain in this treatment modality is seen as the result of an interrupted healing process, so that the pain sufferer is unable to find a place in the world, and is thus unable to remain an integrated person due to ongoing pain experiences. Pain patients, according to this approach, have a deficient organic life and remain in existential need, are angry and distanced from their pain. Therapy therefore aims to return the person to human life by "(re)awakening" through human encounters. The patient in this approach is seen to have "recovered" when they emerge through the encounter as a "whole" person again and does not need a doctor to remain healthy. Finally, the *consciousness* approach provides a further move away from a dualistic framework as "the part of the body which is in pain has become part of here-and-now awareness and has been hurt to the core of existence . . . pain is incorporated into the meaning of being human" (Vrancken 1989: 440). Here, pain patients in principle are anyone complaining of pain and therapy is not specific. Rather, the main prerequisite is the possibility of establishing an interpersonal relationship. This may be any form of treatment but preferably *not* invasive surgery, and the patient is seen to have recovered either when pain disappears or by gaining enough insight to accept and manage it (Vrancken 1989: 436–40).

Vrancken's study suggests an optimistically wide range of possibilities, but whereas integrated multidisciplinary theories may be well developed in the Netherlands, pain clinics in Britain rarely address the phenomenological or consciousness approaches outlined above. However, characteristics of the first three approaches can be readily identified in clinical practice generally and, in particular, in the ethos of the pain clinic in the study here described in this particular chapter. Inevitably, a concentration on, and hierarchical elevation of, the nociceptive or sensory components of pain perception follows, with the result that the neglect or diminishment of the other aspects, particularly the emotional, serves to perpetuate the Cartesian mind/body dualism that is so deeply ingrained in western medicine and culture. As we shall see, it is in this sense that, despite the Foucauldian emphasis upon "biographical" forms of medicine mentioned above, much of contemporary medical practice is still, in fact, firmly rooted in this dualistic legacy.

The implications for the people who experience this particular type of "modern medicine" form the basis of the research described in this chapter, a small-scale qualitative study of a pain relief clinic attached to a teaching hospital in North London. The catchment area had a wide variation in terms of social class, housing, social amenities and ethnicity. Using semistructured interviews, the study explored concepts and beliefs about pain and evaluations of its treatment held by both attenders and staff at the clinics. In keeping with the aims of this volume, however, this particular chapter focuses upon the views of the former, and their responses are analyzed in terms of two broad themes.

The first theme to be considered concerns a description of respondents' past histories and present relationships to pain – that is, their *"pain careers"*. This is important as it has obvious implications in terms of how people perceive and evaluate their treatment (Calnan 1988). Secondly, having looked at people's pain careers, their expectations and evaluation of consultations, management and treatments offered at the pain clinic will then be presented. More generally, a major consideration of the book as a whole is the way in which "medicalization" is seen to impinge upon people's lives. Hence, an overarching theme in this chapter is the extent to which the respondents in this particular study were critical and pro-active with regard to the treatment they received, or simply became passive and accepting of whatever was offered. As Williams (1993) notes, the chronically ill may come to view medicine as both a "fountain of hope and a font of despair", and the aim of this chapter is to assess the extent to which this is also true of chronic pain patients. In doing so, consideration will also be given to the effects of social factors such as age, gender and social class in these processes, although the size of the sample precludes making broad generalizations. Before proceeding to a discussion of these issues, however, a brief sketch of the "ethos of the pain clinic" may provide a useful backdrop to the accounts and evaluations that follow.

The ethos of the pain clinic

There were two pain relief clinics per week under the charge of the consultant anaesthetist. One was for new referrals, held in the out-patient department, and assisted by a senior registrar, a receptionist, a porter and a clinic nurse, who were all regular staff. Up to eight patients were booked in to this clinic at each session, but there were many last-minute cancellations and often as few as three patients appeared for their appointments. Consultations usually involved history taking, treatment plans, and referrals elsewhere if it was felt that the pain relief clinic was inappropriate. In contrast, the second clinic was squeezed into a dormitory of an oncology ward, as there was an ongoing problem of space for out-patient clinics. The consultant expressed the view that this was a reflection of the low priority given to pain patients by the hospital administration. This clinic concentrated on treatment, and was assisted by the same registrar, two clinic nurses who alternated each week, and an acupuncturist, who also ran a private practice outside the hospital. Again a maximum of eight people attended at any session.

The consultant had a sophisticated approach to pain, seeing it as a complex interaction between physical sensations, psychological states and social factors, and felt that the ethos of both clinics was probably best expressed in the dualistic body-orientated approach. In this model, there are three types of pain patients: chronic benign, chronic malignant and chronic pain syndrome (CPS), differentiated by clinical history. If the nociceptive elements are considered intractable, physicians will refer patients to psychologists, incorporating the behaviouristic approach in the form of pain "management", often in separate clinics. Referrals were made to the clinic, and the initial consultation laid great emphasis on the "whole person", taking into account their previous history and present circumstances. At this stage, either a treatment plan was established, involving one or more of the techniques described earlier, or the pain was classed as "intractable" and the pain management clinic was often recommended. The consultant had introduced the use of acupuncture to the clinic, which he regarded as a pioneering attempt to provide an "alternative", more holistic approach to pain relief. However, the acupuncturist expressed severe reservations about these claims as she felt that the inadequacy of resources meant that she had to practise in a way that actually reinforced the dualistic mechanistic model, rather than being able to treat the "whole" person.

Apart from acupuncture, the main forms of treatment administered were interventional nerve blocks (a form of epidural given under local anaesthetic), and analgesics, often narcotics. The health professionals working in the clinic felt that the problem of the lack of economic and practical resources was compounded by the chronicity of the patients' complaints. Despite the intent to create an holistic ethos, attenders were often described by staff in somatico-technical terms that classified them into those with "real pain", "psychiatric disorders" and "malingerers". By the time they reached the pain clinic, the majority of the sample had been through numerous other treatment routes (the consultant described attenders as "lonely despairing people"). Certainly, there was a strong perception among the attenders of the clinic that it represented their "last hope", but this was not borne out by the staff themselves. This role was reserved for the pain management clinic, which provided behaviour therapy to help patients "come to terms" with pain that was unlikely ever to disappear. Pain patients are often seen to have invested their identity in the pain and/or their coping mechanisms are assumed to have "failed". The "ideal" patient, in contrast, can be convinced that their pain is linked to particular situations and is willing to "co-operate" in a programme. Therapy aims to minimize pain behaviour by setting achievable goals such as rehabilitation and resocialization.

Although the pain management clinic was presented to patients as a "viable alternative" (and doubtless did provide a means of trying to cope positively with pain), all the staff expressed ambivalent attitudes in private, often that it was a "dumping ground", as the following examples illustrate:

. . . that's where the real no-hopers go, you should see it, it's like a psychy [psychiatric] ward, they're all spaced out on tranks and anti-depressants, doing OT, making baskets, it's awful. I wouldn't like to work there (female clinic nurse).

It's a harsh fact of life that the majority of cases we get, we can't really help them because they're so chronic and the whole thing has being going on for so long, it's impossible to tell what's going on any more. There's no evident pathology, often there's dependency or addiction to drugs or even alcohol. Then marriages break up because of it, families give up on them because they become so difficult, they have housing problems – by the time they get here, it's not really a medical problem any more, it's more social, but we're expected to pick up the pieces . . . so if we can't cope here, we send them on to [the behaviour therapy] clinic, it's more geared up for all that there (male registrar).

This hierarchical relegation of conditions and treatments that are concerned with psychological and emotional states serves to perpetuate the Cartesian split between mind and body and clearly illustrates how the notion of "cure" elevates the status of pain with a demonstrable, preferably physiological component (see Bendelow 1993, Bendelow & Williams 1995 for a fuller discussion). Not surprisingly, as we shall see, these attitudes were picked up and reflected in the responses of patients themselves.

Everyone who attended the clinics over the period of fieldwork lasting two months, was approached to take part in the interviews, and of these 42 men and women, eight declined to take part in the study. Most of the interviews took place at the Wednesday clinics, after the treatment session. Demographic details such as age, sex, occupation, ethnicity and housing circumstances were collected. Altogether, ten women and two men were under 40, six men and six women were aged between 40 and 60, and eight women and four men were aged 60 and over. A striking factor is that there were twice as many women attending the clinics as there were men (including the respondents who refused to take part). Using the Registrar General's classification of occupations, 60 per cent (20) of the sample were classified as "working class" or unemployed, and the remaining 40 per cent had "middle-class" occupations. Out of the whole sample, only two men and four women defined themselves as other than "white UK or Irish born", being either Pakistani, Iranian or Greek Cypriot.

Pain "careers"

As mentioned earlier, nearly all the respondents in the sample had received or pursued various forms of treatment, apart from consulting their GP, in order to alleviate their pain. The only person who had been referred directly to the clinic by her GP was an Iranian woman, a refugee, in very extreme circumstance.[1] All the sample had used various forms of analgesics, and 25 used painkillers every day. Twenty-eight people had tried physiotherapy and ten had consulted an osteopath or chiropractor. The use of other treatments also related to the length of time that the respondent had suffered from pain, which varied from six months to 23 years, the average time being seven years. The most important factor here was age, but not only was old age associated with more years of pain, it was also the case that the younger the person, the less time they had to wait for a referral to the clinic. Indeed, none of respondents in the younger age groups (20–30 and 30–40 years) had been in pain longer than a year before being referred and, on the whole, men appeared to have been referred sooner than women. Although just over a third (12) of the sample could not attribute any original incident or cause for the pain, the remaining 22 claimed the pain was a result of an initial physical trauma or accident, such as the following: a fracture, a fall as a result of a chair being pulled away and an accident using a chainsaw. However, in the majority of these cases (18), there was no residual pathology or tissue damage. In other words although physiologically speaking, the body had healed, pain was still being experienced. As regards the bodily location of the pain, over half the sample (20) had pain in the back or abdomen and five complained of pain in the leg, usually the knee. Three people had pain in their upper limbs, four had recurrent violent headaches and one man had continual pain in his right hand and right testicle.

When the respondents were invited to take part in the interviews, it was emphasized that their own feelings about what was happening to them were the central focus of the study, rather than a formal clinical account. Interestingly, most respondents expressed surprise that anyone would be "bothered" to seek this information, but were pleased rather than wary with the result that many of the interviews were very open and revealing. Everyone who was interviewed felt without doubt that as well as the physical limitations, pain had a very negative emotional effect, ranging from irritability to depression, with inevitable consequences for self-esteem, confidence and social relationships. However, there were differences in attitudes towards the overall effect on people's lives that could be divided into two broad categories. Generally the first group expressed the feeling that their lives were totally dominated by the pain (cf. Herzlich's (1973) "illness as destroyer"), in that there was no hope for the future, as the pain, it was thought, would never disappear. In other words, this group displayed classic features of *resignation*. That is to say, those who

> (i) dwell upon their condition (ii) feel psychologically cut off or isolated from others (iii) feel hopeless or depressed as a result of their condition (iv) indicate that they are missing out on social activities in which they previously engaged, or which are enjoyed by other people (v) express directly the view that illness has come to dominate their life (Radley & Green 1987: 190).

In this sense, modern medicine, in the form of the pain clinic, represents the only possible means of salvation in the hope of finding a "cure". Referring back to Kotarba's three stage theory of chronic pain adjustment, this group of people can be described as having emerged through the first two stages into the "chronic pain career". However, rather than displaying a simplistic "blanket dependence", this group also expressed cynicism and ambivalence as to whether, in the end, medicine could actually be of any real help to their plight.

This chronic pain sequence was also true of most of the respondents in the second group, but there were marked differences in their styles of adjustment. Although they felt the quality of their lives had been severely affected, they could still nonetheless envisage a "pain-free" future. Although this group could be seen to employ elements of an *active denial* strategy, seeing their life as a battle against pain, they more often expressed what Radley & Green (1987) refer to as an *accommodative* style of adjustment, incorporating pain into their lives and adjusting to it in a more positive manner. For this group, their attendance at the clinic played an important but not central role.

Sadly the first group, which I shall refer to in this chapter as the "resignation group" was the larger of the two, comprising nine men and 12 women (62 per cent of the total sample). In contrast, the remaining 38 per cent of the sample (three males and ten females) formed what I shall term the "accommodation group".

Suicidal ideas and thoughts were expressed frankly by 20 interviewees, with similar numbers of men and women voicing these feelings. Perhaps not surprisingly, this severe despair was expressed by most of the people in the "resignation" group. Within this group, most people (18) felt there was no distraction from the pain, and, beyond the treatment offered by the clinic, most (19) saw painkillers or alcohol as the most effective means of coping with it. All these respondents complained of feeling socially isolated, even from family members or people they lived with, and nearly two-thirds (13) lived alone, often as a result of the break-up of a marriage or cohabiting relationship. Pain dominated their lives totally, and nearly all of them (19) expressed notions of self-blame regarding their predicament. The following quotes illustrate how despairing some of these respondents felt:

> I can't describe how it's destroyed me. Ten years ago, before all this began, I was a teacher, we'd just got married, buying our own house, the fairy story you know. Now I've got nothing. I had to give up my job, my husband went off with someone else two years ago, he couldn't stand my whining any longer. We had to sell the house and I live in a rat-hole of a flat. I have to climb two flights of stairs 'cos there's no lift. Most nights if I'm honest I spend watching TV and drinking enough to blot it all out. If it wasn't for my friend who still comes over, I'd quite happily do myself in. I know I shouldn't say that, but what's there to live for? (female, unemployed, aged 35).

> My life is just hell, complete misery, I don't know why someone can't just put me down, if it was a dog it wouldn't suffer . . . and these bloody doctors, I could swing for them, I don't know why they can't find out what causes it. I can't do my job for the pain in my belly, I'm just about to be made redundant and I bet I'll lose my pension. The wife and kids are fed up with me moaning and yelling at them all the time. The only pleasure I've got is the bloody whisky and beer, but of course they tell you off and say I've to stop smoking. I've had the big intestine cut four times you see. It's all very well for them, that's all I've got . . . (male, school caretaker, aged 58).

> All I do is go to work, type all day, then come back to my mum and dad, take more tablets and watch telly. I don't go out any more, I just sit and think, why did it happen, why did that boy pull out the chair from under me, why me? I must be bad for that to happen, I can't help it, it's all I can think about . . . (female, clerical worker, aged 21).

In contrast, the other "accommodation" group were able to distract themselves from their pain, by using physical or intellectual activities, hobbies or work. Their coping mechanisms included painkillers and alcohol on occasion, but they also used a variety of other resources, which could be physical, such as comfort or heat, or emotional, such as social support from partners, children, relatives and friends:

> I would like to think that one day it'll go away but I know that maybe it won't. Whenever it gets really, really, bad I try to be

warm, comfortable, sometimes I just have to give in and I say to the kids, "come and cuddle Mummy" and they are so sweet, Jody's only four and I lie there with tears streaming down my face and she wipes them away, but we laugh as well and Jim, my husband, will give me a massage and muck about. It's not all as awful as all that. Or I'll be really strong and just say I'm going to ignore it and take them to the park, feed the ducks, anything to distract me . . . (female full-time mother, aged 32).

Well, I use work a lot, I find it really helps to get so distracted. It doesn't go away exactly but somehow it's more bearable . . . (male, self-employed architect, aged 45).

At my age I know I'll probably never get rid of it, but what do I do? I play the piano, that's the best thing for it! (male, retired Naval Officer, aged 75).

When the two groups were compared, the most obvious differences were in pain chronicity, so that people in the resignation group were more likely to have been in pain for a longer period of time. Yet other social factors, particularly social class also appeared to mediate here. In this respect, notably more "middle-class" patients tended to be in the second, more hopeful group, although not exclusively so.

Poor housing and lack of social support, especially for those living alone, appeared to be contributory factors to the desperation and hopelessness of the first group. Some of these people had grown up in very different cultures, such as those of Pakistani or Irish origin, and felt very vulnerable to the harsh reality of inner city living. For example, an elderly Greek Cypriot man described how his depression over his back pain was compounded by his exile from his country. He thought that there would be much more to live for if he could only sit in the sunshine on his veranda in the house he had to leave 20 years ago.

When asked what helped the most, aside from medical treatment, in terms of coping with chronic pain, there also appeared to be gender differences. For men, occupational status and material advantages, particularly the ability to maintain their income level, were seen as the most important factors, with the subsequent implications of "failure" when these were lost. In contrast, whereas these aspects were also important for the women in the sample, social support was perceived to be of equal importance.

Experiences of the pain clinic

Treatment for pain relief was seen by many in the "resignation" group literally as that, as the following two examples of respondents with low back pain demonstrate:

> Eight years I've had this pain . . . I've been through everything you could possibly think of trying to get to the bottom of this. My GP told me I was imagining it, that I was being neurotic because the kids had left home. He sent me for X-rays, all sorts of specialists, nothing worked. I even tried an osteopath, that was useless . . . I'd given up completely, just lived on painkillers . . . then I got the appointment for here. I couldn't believe it, it's the only place that's taken me seriously . . . (female, aged 48, ex-florist, now supported by husband).

> That Dr G – he's wonderful, he really listens to you and takes everything into account, I'm so happy to be coming here, I can't believe it. All the other doctors, they made me feel, you know, like I was making it up and I were rubbish, I didn't think I'd ever get nothing, no help. Now he's going to try me with these block things, it's like someone believes me after five years of hell, it's the light at the end of the tunnel . . . (female, retired machinist, aged 66).

There was a tendency, especially among the female attenders in this group, to place high expectations on the treatment generally, and the consultant in particular, to provide a "miracle cure". In most cases, the interview took place after the treatment session, and the more recently this had been instigated, the more effective the response. The following reactions were given by two women who had just received their first session of nerve blocks:

> I was so scared at first, the sight of those great big needles, I nearly passed out I was that scared, but I have to say I think it worked . . . nothing else ever has apart from the painkillers. I'm at a stage where I've given up on anything really, I couldn't see any point in coming here or in anything really, but if this, if the feeling lasts then it's a miracle . . . (female, living alone on benefit, aged 40).

> It sounds horrendous, doesn't it, you'd never usually agree to something like that but they're so kind and patient, they explain it all, what they're doing and it really has made it go away, I'm too scared to believe it, I've been out of my mind with it, totally

desperate. I said to my boyfriend, just tell them to put me to sleep. But this is incredible, I think this place is wonderful! (Female, student, aged 21).

Another woman, who described her life as a "total disaster" had been the recipient of nerve block treatment in sessions of three months at a time for over five years. She relied heavily on painkillers, and also used food as a source of comfort, with the result that, at 20 stones, she was extremely overweight; something that increased her misery still further. In the interview, she claimed that the treatment sessions were all that she lived for, and that her life in between treatments was completely empty, despite the support of her two teenage children and husband, who all accompanied her to the clinic. Usually, treatment with nerve blocks was not given beyond a year, as the consultant claimed the efficacy appeared to diminish over time. However, his rationale for continuing in this particular case was that there was, in fact, some "placebo effect".

In contrast, the males in the "resignation" group did not appear to hold such high expectations of treatment, and perceived their attendance at the clinic much more negatively as being the "end of the line":

Well, they don't know what else to do with me do they? That's why I'm here so they can stick needles in me, experiment. Like I'm no good for nothing else am I? (male, ex-HGV driver, aged 51).

Indeed, six people in this group were advised during their appointment that the clinic was unable to offer appropriate treatment. Five of these respondents were women, four of whom had waited many months for the appointment, seeing it very much, as described above, as their last hope. These people all expressed great disappointment and a sense of personal failure at not being offered any of the treatments available in the clinic. They also all expressed much resentment at being referred to the pain management clinic, interpreting it as "second-rate" treatment and echoing the views of the clinic staff described earlier:

I just can't cope with it, I mean I had such high hopes of coming here, that finally they'd make me better. I don't want to learn to *manage* it, I want to get *rid* of it. Now I just feel I might as well give up, it's going to be there for the rest of my life . . . (female, shop assistant, aged 33).

All these women spent some of the interview in tears, as did the fifth woman who had been advised that her course of nerve blocks would not be continued:

> I just wish I'd lied and said they were working, that the pain had gone. I just feel like they've given up on me here, sending me to that other place [the pain management clinic]. I've heard bad things about that . . . (female, living alone on benefit, aged 57).

The one male who was turned down for treatment in the clinic was referred directly to a psychiatrist, much to his disgust. He described numerous violent incidents in his past history, resulting in various stabbings and other injuries, which he claimed accounted for the pains in his finger, stomach and right testicle, but no trauma could be found. Additionally, his appearance and manner were quite alarming, a huge, multi-tattooed man who was verbally abusive and apparently had physically threatened the consultant. He became extremely angry during the interview as he recounted his story, and eventually stormed out, shouting his opinions as to his diagnosis at the receptionist, who became very agitated and called security to ensure he was kept off the premises!

Of the remaining 28 people in the sample, roughly half (15) were receiving acupuncture as a treatment, and nearly all these respondents could be categorized into the more optimistic "accommodation" group discussed earlier. However, the three women and one man in the "resignation group" who were receiving acupuncture felt it gave them no relief and indicated that they thought it was a "complete waste of time". For instance:

> It's a complete waste of time, if you really want to know. I don't know why I bother coming. You might as well start saying magic spells or do some voodoo. I don't know, it's all a big con but I don't like to tell her, she's such a nice lady. I was so pleased about coming here, I can't tell you, but I'm still in as much pain as ever . . . (female, retired machinist, aged 62).

In common with the others in the "resignation" group who were mostly receiving nerve blocks or narcotics, they saw their pain as somatic, needing physical intervention and appeared to be expecting medicine in this clinic to provide the "miracle cure", often after many years of waiting. When the treatment "failed", either by not providing relief, or more usually, providing only temporary relief as in the case of nerve blocks, they felt totally despondent. Although, on the one hand, this group could be described as being critical of modern medical techniques, it could also be argued that this was partly due to their rather unrealistic expectations, given the nature and chronicity of their condition. In this way, their reliance on medicine to find the answers created an over-dependence and passivity, which was often undermined by many years of mismanagement concerning their condition.

In contrast, the "accommodation" group could be seen to have a much wider, more integrated view of the effect of chronic pain on their lives, which was itself a strong indicator for being "prescribed" acupuncture. Although, as described earlier, the acupuncturist herself had grave reservations about the limitations of her practice in the clinic, all the recipients in this group spoke enthusiastically about her holistic approach:

> She really makes you feel like she's interested in you as a whole person, that all sorts of things in your life are important and can affect how you feel, she explains all this while she puts the needles in and you feel so sort of . . . I don't know . . . looked after that you don't feel any pain when she puts them in. Maybe that's how it works! I don't know that it makes it go away exactly, but I always feel better, somehow, more able to deal with it . . . (female, housing officer, aged 34).

> I was really suspicious at first when he told me I'd be having acupuncture, I thought it was a bit quackish, you know, but I have to say, she's really good. I'd never really thought how much stress and things like that could play a part in something like this, and she explains it all, takes your own personal history into account, it's amazing, it's converted me, it really helps the pain. I must admit though, that first time when she put a needle in here, in the belly, I thought "Jesus Christ, what have I let myself in for!" it was bad enough down the leg! (male, unemployed architect, aged 53).

> It's just the most incredible sensation, she puts the needles in the arms, the legs, one in the forehead, one in the groin, yes that's a bit unnerving, but they're very thin you see, you can hardly feel them. Then you get this sort of electrical charge buzzing round all the needles, right through your body, which she explains it's sort of like psychic energy that's released which has pain killing properties . . . (female, ex dance-teacher, aged 45).

For this group, therefore, attendance at the clinic and treatment are a part and parcel of a broader strategy of coping, which is not simply dependent on the biomedical concept of cure, but has resonances with more holistic approaches (such as the *phenomenological* and *consciousness* approaches described earlier by Vrancken (1989)) that integrate mind and body and see medicine as a part rather than the whole of the healing process.

Discussion

In order to explore the lay experience of chronic pain, Bazanger (1989) has stressed the use of a phenomenological approach, and has applauded the attempts within medical sociology to enquire into the connotations of "living with" illness and the experience of the sufferer. She maintains that this process results in illness becoming "free of medicine", restoring it to the patient; something that, she suggests, is a welcome reaction to the "medicocentrism" of earlier theorists such as Parsons (1951). Similarly, Kotarba (1983) has emphasized how, with respect to the "chronic pain career" two themes emerge – the clinical and the experiential. These themes, in turn, relate to Mishler's (1984) delineation of the struggle between the "voice of medicine" (i.e. biomedical and clinical) and the "voice of the lifeworld" (i.e. biographical, social and contextual); a situation that is echoed in the data presented in this particular study. Although these experiences may not be mutually exclusive, there is nonetheless a hierarchy in which the former is often assumed to be routine and normative whereas the latter is frequently perceived to be at worst irrelevant, and at best disruptive.

Yet as other writers have similarly argued (Gabe & Calnan 1989, Kohler Riessman 1989, Calnan & Williams 1992), the data also suggest that, although doctors may indeed create dependence in their patients, to portray them simply as passive and accepting on the one hand, or as independent and pro-active on the other, may be misleading and overly simplistic. Indeed, as this study clearly shows, although the larger "resignation" group of attenders were the more dependent on the techniques of modern medicine, they were also more dissatisfied, critical and undermined by their experiences. Whether this would be the case irrespective of the treatment they received in this particular clinic is, however, difficult to decipher as these experience are so closely tied to their own personal biographies and narratives. In contrast, the more independent "accommodation" group who appeared more highly motivated, and thus more "acceptable" to clinicians, were more likely to be satisfied and to express positive experiences of their treatment. Nonetheless, despite these differences, pain was viewed unambiguously as a negative experience for both groups, although in differing degrees, and there is nothing in the data to suggest Herzlich's final category (1973) of "illness as liberator".

The most important factor in differentiating between these two groups appeared to be the chronicity of the condition. Many people had spent years in pain, and experienced a variety of therapies, but had often been made to feel a nuisance, especially when no physiological basis for the pain was found. This continual lowering of self-esteem appeared to have as much, if not more, impact as the physical limitations, resulting in inextricable emotional and psychiatric features of the condition.

Regarding socio-demographic characteristics, age was clearly important here, in that younger people had often spent less time in pain and, in this study at least, appeared to have been more quickly referred for treatment. In addition, social class also appeared to play a role in that middle-class respondents seemed to be more likely to accommodate pain in their lives, and to try various strategies to positively "manage" it. In contrast, lower occupational status, especially when combined with social isolation and poor housing, was associated with a sense of hopelessness, despair and suicidal wishes.

Turning to gender, as other studies have similarly found (Csordas & Clark 1992), the high number of women attenders at this clinic is not unusual. When asked why they thought there were twice as many female as male attenders, all the staff expressed the view in some form or other that women were more likely to perceive themselves to be in pain, especially if the pain was psychological in origin, and that they were more likely to report it and "give in" to it, letting it dominate their lives. It may be the case that as women are perceived to complain more, men are taken more seriously – as we saw, the only man to be turned away for treatment was perceived as very threatening and needing psychiatric treatment. Yet, while the professionals were inclined to perceive women as more likely to adopt a fatalistic "sick role", this was not borne out by the data. Moreover, there were also gender differences regarding factors perceived as being important in "coping" with pain, in that men tended to stress occupational and material status, whereas women were likely to place greater emphasis upon social support. Clearly, however, given the small-scale nature of this study, broader generalizations cannot be made, although these findings are instructive.

Another important factor in these experiences of modern medicine appears to be the impact of the mind/body dualism in the approach to treatment. On the whole, the ethos of the clinic appeared to perpetuate the dualism in the sense that the attenders in the "resignation" category were anxious for their pain to be viewed as "real", which meant conceptualizing their pain in somatic terms. As a consequence, they often expressed extreme despair if no physical pathology could be found. Alternatively, those in the "accommodation" group appeared to feel less stigmatized and less defensive about being in chronic pain. Subsequently, more positive reports of treatment tended to be associated with the more integrated holistic approach of acupuncture than the "somatico-technical" interventional nerve blocks. In this respect, it is instructive to note that most of the highly motivated "accommodation" group were receiving the former type of treatment.

To conclude, unless very highly motivated and thus conforming to their stereotype of the "ideal patient", pain clinic staff on the whole tended to perceive their patients as complex, chronic and "low-status", with little chance of being able to be helped. These attitudes were in turn absorbed and reflected in the perceptions of those receiving the treatments, evoking a striking resemblance to the grim situation described some two decades ago by Anslem Strauss (1973) in his classic book *Where medicine fails*.

Furthermore, the use of a qualitative and interpretative approach enabled respondents to discuss frankly their feelings and emotions in their evaluations of the treatments offered, revealing varying degrees of ambiguity and complexity. Undoubtedly the ultimate goal for the majority of the recipients of treatment in the pain relief clinic was a "pain free" existence, but unfortunately this was something that was rarely achieved due to the nature of the chronic pain syndrome. Whereas a number of attenders were able to view their treatment as a positive experience, and to see it as one of a range of resources they used to "manage" their pain, the majority expressed varying degrees of disappointment, frustration and disillusionment. In many cases, years had been spent in chronic pain and the expectations of the clinic to provide a "last ditch" cure were very high. Unfortunately, given this combination of a high degree of anticipation and the limitations of current medical techniques, the all too common feeling of people in this study was that medicine was "failing" them.

Notes

1. This woman had fled from Iran in 1991 having suffered imprisonment and torture which she attributed as the cause of her back pain.

References

Armstrong, D. 1983. *Political anatomy of the body*. Cambridge: Cambridge University Press.

Arney, W. R. & J. Neill 1983. The location of pain in childbirth. *Sociology of Health and Illness* **7**, 109–17.

Bazanger, I. 1989. Pain: its experience and treatment. *Social Science and Medicine* **29**(3), 425–34.

Bendelow, G. 1993. Pain perceptions, emotion and gender. *Sociology of Health and Illness* **15**(3), 273–9.

Bendelow, G. & S. J. Williams 1995. Transcending the dualisms: towards a sociology of pain. *Sociology of Health and Illness* **17**(2), 139–65.

Bonica, J. 1953. The management of pain. Philadelphia: Lea & Febiger.

Bury, M. 1982. Chronic illness as biographical disruption. *Sociology of Health*

REFERENCES

and Illness **4**, 167–82.

Bury, M. 1991. The sociology of chronic illness: a review of research and prospects. *Sociology of Health and Illness* **13**(4), 451–68.

Calnan, M. 1988. Toward a conceptual framework of lay evaluation of health care. *Social Science and Medicine* **27**(9), 927–33.

Calnan, M. & S. J. Williams 1992. Images of scientific medicine. *Sociology of Health and Illness* **14**(2), 233–54.

Csordas, T. & J. Clark 1992. Ends of the line: diversity among chronic pain centers. *Social Science and Medicine* **34**(4), 383–93.

Gabe, J. & M. Calnan 1989. The limits of medicine: women's perception of medical technology. *Social Science and Medicine* **28**(3), 223–31.

Herzlich, C. 1973. *Health and illness: a social psychological approach*. New York: Academic Press.

Kohler Riessman, C. 1989. Women and medicalization: a new perspective. In *Perspectives in medical sociology*, P. Brown (ed.), 190–220. Belmont, California: Wadsworth.

Kotarba, J. 1983. *Chronic pain: its social dimensions*. Beverly Hills, California: Sage.

Melzack, R. & P. Wall 1988. *The challenge of pain*. London: Penguin.

Mishler, H. 1984. *The discourse of medicine*. Cambridge: Cambridge University Press.

Nettleton, S. 1992. *Power, pain & dentistry*. Milton Keynes: Open University Press.

Parsons, T. 1951. *The social system*. London: Routledge & Kegan Paul.

Radley, A. & R. Green 1987. Illness as adjustment: a methodology and conceptual framework. *Sociology of Health and Illness* **9**(2), 179–207.

Sarafino E. 1991. *Health psychology: a biopsychosocial approach*. Beverly Hills, California: Sage.

Saunders, C. 1976. Care of the dying. *Nursing Times* **72**, 3–24.

Strauss, A. 1973. *Where medicine fails*. New Brunswick, New Jersey: Transaction Books.

Vrancken, M. 1989. Schools of thought on pain. *Social Science and Medicine* **29**(3), 435–44.

Williams, D. & B. Thorn 1989. An empirical assessment of pain beliefs. *Pain* **36**, 351–8.

Williams, G. 1984. The genesis of chronic illness: narrative reconstruction. *Sociology of Health and Illness* **6**(2), 175–200.

Williams, S. J. 1993. *Chronic respiratory illness*. London: Routledge.

Part IV

Women and reproductive technology

Chapter 9

Pain and pain relief in labour: issues of control

Lynda Rajan

Introduction

Pain is generally viewed as something to be avoided at all cost. While its value as a physiological phenomenon is acknowledged, in that it signals dysfunction, disease or trauma, at the same time it is disruptive and detrimental to normal functioning. Childbirth is one of the few occasions in which pain is the acceptable manifestation of a normal process. The pain of labour is productive pain, usually with a tangible outcome, the baby, and certainly with a finite course that ends with the delivery of the placenta. If it is a first baby it marks the beginning of the woman's status as a mother; if she has other children it brings a new dimension to other relationships within the family. In any case, the birth precipitates a radical change in the woman's life. Thus the pain that she experiences in labour has a different meaning to her from other types of pain. It is legitimate to ask, therefore, whether the wider implications of that experience of pain also differ, and if so, in what ways?

This chapter seeks to address issues of medicalization, power and control in relation to women's experiences of pain and pain relief in childbirth. Are women active or passive? Are they in control or dependent? And to what extent does the technology employed serve to liberate or alienate them from their bodies?

Medicalization, childbirth and the "problem" of medical technology

The medicalization of the birth process has resulted in an increased reliance on drugs and technology as a means of managing this pain, to such an extent that it has transformed the meaning of childbirth from a normal healthy human experience to a problem that requires medical intervention as the norm (Kohler Riessman 1983). One consequence of this for the pregnant woman is that by viewing birth as "abnormal", and being obliged to seek medical assistance, she automatically surrenders autonomy and thereby assumes a subordinate role in the process. In doing so, she literally loses control of her body and self for the duration of the labour.

Certainly it is clear, as we edge ever closer to the twenty-first century, that a panoply of technology now pervades the field of reproduction. As Stanworth (1987) argues, this can usefully be grouped into four main categories. First, fertility controls such at the pill, diaphragms, intra-uterine devices (IUDs) and condoms; secondly, those designed to "manage" labour and childbirth such as foetal monitoring, episiotomies, Caesarean sections and the use of forceps; thirdly, screening techniques such as ultrasound and amniocentesis designed to detect foetal "defects"; and finally, newer forms of technology that are designed to overcome infertility. In short, from their historical position as "birth helpers" or "attendants", in which "Nature" was seen to be the controlling force, obstetricians and midwives have now become "birth controllers", curbing "Nature" itself through these differing forms of technological intervention.

In recent years, however, a new movement has evolved, in which women have tried to regain their autonomy in childbirth by "de-medicalizing" the process. In this respect, the call for home births, involvement in support groups like the National Childbirth Trust, and the use of "alternative" methods of pain relief, such as aromatherapy, homeopathy and acupuncture have all increased. Yet as Arney & Neill (1983) have argued, this shift from a one to a two-dimensional conception of pain in childbirth may actually serve to increase medical power and control through the incorporation of patient subjectivity into the web of medical surveillance that surrounds and pervades women's bodies and minds. Moreover, as Kohler Riessman (1983) has argued, women have not simply been passive victims of medical technology. Rather, they have actively collaborated in the medicalization process in order to satisfy their own needs and motives, which in turn derive from their subordinate social position and their class-related interests. In this sense, as Lupton (1994) has recently argued, far from simply being "oppressive", medical technology may actually serve as a "resource" in women's lives and a means of "liberation" from the constraints of their embodiment (see also Chapter 10). Furthermore, as Gabe & Calnan (1989) suggest, there may be two types of woman: the active consumer who takes control of the technology available and uses it according to need, and the passive user of whatever is on offer because no choice is perceived to be available – though even the latter may draw on other resources to help them cope. Certainly, as Evans (1985) suggests, women are ambivalent about medical technology, on the one hand expressing a desire for more control over their pregnancies, while on the other hand, simultaneously expressing a desire for more medical technology.

The feminist movement, in requiring women to question their subordination, has empowered them to seek out other resources and alternative means of regaining and retaining control over the birth process, as well as to take a critical view of the "benefits" of technological interventions (Oakley 1984). These other resources, including "alternative" pain relief methods, play a crucial role and are valued by women due to the absence of side-effects both for themselves and their babies. The deleterious impact of pharmacological methods on the baby's neurological state, on its ability to feed, and on her own efforts to initiate and sustain breast-feeding is often a vital consideration for the mother in deciding against their use. Yet "alternative" methods may represent to the medical profession a rejection of their own skills and technologies, and hence of their own role in the process of birth.

Studies of approaches to pain relief

The evaluation of the need for and the effectiveness of analgesia is thus a complex subject that must include assessment of issues other than the level of pain per se, both in general (Bendelow 1992) and during labour and delivery (Simkin 1989, Dickersin 1989). It also raises issues of control. Other studies have shown a lack of convergence in people's perceptions of the same experience of pain, and the systematic undertreatment with narcotics of medical patients, especially those with terminal illnesses (Marks & Sachar 1973, McCaffery & Hart 1976, Melzack 1990). Gynaecological ward nurses have been shown to overestimate patients' worries while underestimating the duration and intensity of pain (Johnston 1976). Bradley et al. (1983) suggested that this tendency might be a result of stereotyped thinking by nurses who do not know their patients well, and speculated that midwives' more prolonged and intimate contact with labouring women should enable them to judge the amount of pain experienced more accurately, though this was not borne out by his research.

In one study of the use of narcotic analgesia in the relief of post-operative pain (Cohen 1980), nurses were found to have other agendas that influenced their actions, as well as an inadequate knowledge of the palliative effect of drugs. Many indicated that complete pain relief was not their major goal, and concern about the possibility of addiction – even with dying patients – caused them to give smaller quantities of drugs than were prescribed by the doctors, or were of use to the patient. Nurses tended to select the lowest of the range of choices available, even if this did not produce the desired effect, the relief of pain. Many nurses were observed to wait for patients to request medication, which caused Cohen to wonder if the patients realized this, or if they relied on the nurses' assessment as to when it would be needed. Value judgements and disapproval often influenced the attitude with which pain relief was given.

Poor communication between professionals and women and the resultant lack of information has been found to cause a great deal of distress and unnecessary worry (Bradley et al. 1983, Rajan 1992, Kirke 1980a,b). Kirke (1980a), for example, found that women who were not satisfied with the care they received in labour rarely questioned the technical competence of professionals attending them, but were very critical of the manner in which the care was provided. Issues of information and control are also significant factors in women's assessment of their own satisfaction with pain relief methods (Green et al. 1988, Morgan et al. 1982). Indeed, Cartwright (1987) identified a "glaring gap" in professionals' knowledge of the outcome of childbirth, including staff ignorance of women's true feelings about their experiences of treatment during labour and the paucity of information and support provided.

One attempt by a consultant obstetrician (Drew et al. 1989) to combat this criticism only succeeded in adding to the evidence that midwives used stereotypes, "albeit accurate ones", in perceiving women's needs, and reflected their tendency both to perceive "average" needs and to impose these when assessing the real needs of individual women. The weakness of the paper is expressed, unwittingly, by Drew himself, when he explains that "purely subjective features were not included; all items were, in principle, objectively identifiable" (p. 1085). Yet it is those very subjective issues that, albeit less easily quantifiable, observable, or rankable, are the essence of the woman's experience of childbirth. By removing "idiosyncratic" and "subjective" items from the list drawn up during preliminary interviews, Drew ensured that the women to whom he then gave the questionnaire were constrained in their responses to talk about ideal practical routines. Thus his results gave only a limited impression of the issues that are really involved.

The present chapter derives from data collected by the National Birthday Trust Fund (NBTF) Pain Relief in Labour study. The NBTF survey was carried out on a sample of all births in one week in 1990 in the UK. Its primary aim was to provide a national picture of the facilities, effectiveness and implications for women and babies of different methods of obstetric analgesia and anaesthesia. The original data were collected from 10,352 women in 293 maternity units. A follow-up postal questionnaire was completed by around 10 per cent of the women six weeks after delivery ($N = 1,149$). This questionnaire contained open-ended questions and a comments section from which the qualitative data in this chapter were derived.

The study originally enabled examination of the so-called "objective" measures of obstetric process and outcome. These are discussed elsewhere (Chamberlain et al. 1993). In addition, the data made it possible to compare those measures with perceptions of subjective issues such as experience versus observation of pain and the effectiveness of anaesthesia between the study women and the midwives, obstetricians, general practitioners and anaesthetists that attended them (Rajan 1993, 1994). For the purposes of the present chapter, however, the extensive qualitative data obtained from the survey allowed insights into the experience of labour pain and anaesthesia and women's impressions of staff attitudes and behaviour, enabling examination of issues such as the impact of social support, power and control, and differing perceptions of the same labour experience.

It could, of course, be argued that such data are not qualitative in the strict sense, in that they are restricted by the format of the questionnaire and limited by its source, scope and content. However, previous research has shown (Oakley 1992) that women often take advantage of the opportunity offered by such surveys to unburden themselves, to express opinions, and to relate relevant life experiences, sometimes at considerable length. Certainly in the NBTF survey follow-up, more than two-fifths of the women felt moved to do so. All too often, because the remit of such a study is to generate quantitative data, such comments cannot be utilized. Yet the value of qualitative data from a study of this kind is that it often goes beyond the confines of the questions asked and brings to the researchers' attention issues that are felt to be important for the women themselves. One of the aims of this part of the secondary analysis was, therefore, to recognize the value of such data and to evaluate their contribution to our understanding of women's experience of labour. Despite its contextual limitations, it can be argued that the very act of responding in this way is an effort to regain some control and exert influence over the medicalized process of childbirth. In this respect, it may perhaps be helpful to conceptualize qualitative data on a continuum ranging from social survey data through to ethnography, provided the limitations of the former are acknowledged.

Perceptions of pain relief and issues of control

As the preceding discussion suggests, the medical management of pain in childbirth raises a number of critical issues surrounding the ownership and control of women's bodies, and the extent to which modern technology constitutes another form of oppression or a potential means of liberation.

One of the findings that clearly emerged from the study was that women and health professionals seemed to hold differing concepts of what actually constituted methods of pain relief. For example, anaesthetists rarely mentioned breathing and relaxation or any "alternative" method as pain relieving, instead confining their attention to pharmacological methods. Obstetricians showed a similar tendency, while just under one-tenth of midwives referred to non-pharmacological methods. This contrasted markedly with women's perceptions: nearly one-third of them mentioned that they had used "alternative" methods of pain relief. Hence, the following discussion is structured in order to reflect this division between "conventional" and "alternative" methods of pain relief and the issues of power and control it raises in women's lives.

"Conventional" pharmacological methods of pain relief

While 6 per cent of the women had planned to use no pain relief at all, only 3 per cent actually ended up doing so. Many of the latter, however, had not intended to do without, as the following quote testifies:

> I did not have any pain relief. When I entered the delivery room I asked for an epidural but was told the anaesthetist was in the operating theatre. I was not happy with that matter but there was little I could do.

Entonox, or "gas and air", was the most commonly used method of pain relief. While midwives tended not to consider it particularly helpful on the whole, women in contrast, regarded it more highly. This apparent paradox may derive from the fact that, although a pharmacological method, Entonox is one that women administer themselves. Unlike TENS (Transcutaneous Electrical Nerve Stimulation), it is almost universally provided, but women can decide whether or not to use it at any stage of labour. The only influence a member of staff can have over its use is not to inform the woman of its existence on the labour ward, or to advise against its use, as apparently happened here:

> I was not offered TENS or gas and air as the midwife explained later that she did not think I needed them.

Where they are aware of its availability, women may regard Entonox as part of their "armoury" and be empowered by the relief it gives, however limited that may be, because it is within their own control, as these women explained:

When she told me about the Entonox it was the greatest relief in the world. My husband was massaging my back and I felt like I was floating, totally high.

I had pethidine and gas and air in two previous labours and I didn't feel I was in control at all, so this time I just had the gas and air. I felt much more in control and didn't notice the pain was any worse.

The only pain relief in labour was Entonox which was adequate, easily controlled by myself and helped tremendously.

Some women, however, expressed mixed feelings about the method, and a few gave very negative comments:

I only had gas and air as my labour was too quick for anything else. It didn't help me at all, whereas with my first child it helped me 100 per cent. But I think the reason was that my labour was too quick for my body to cope with.

I don't know if the gas and air made any difference to my pain relief because it made me so aggressive and scared. It made me so high that half the time I did not know where I was or what was happening to me . . . I also did not listen to what I was being told to do – the end result was that I tore and had to have stitches. It was not a nice feeling at all.

We can hear, in this last comment, a sad echo of the power relationship embedded within that labour, almost as if having to have stitches was considered "retribution" for "disobedience".

Of all methods of pain relief, apart from the general anaesthetic (which was regarded by the women more as a surgical procedure than a method of pain relief), epidural anaesthesia renders the woman the most helpless. Yet paradoxically for many women, its efficacy in giving complete freedom from pain enabled them to retain a sense of "control" over other aspects of their labour, even when, as for the second of the two women below, its use was not in accordance with the woman's original birth plan:

For me the epidural worked perfectly. I dozed through most of the birth and I could wriggle my toes and lift my legs. When I was fully dilated the epidural had just worn off enough to make it uncomfortable, so I was able to push my baby out without the need of forceps.

I had been hoping and planning for a "natural" childbirth with minimal intervention. The severity of the pain during my first stage was such that I needed an epidural. I was disappointed to have had so much intervention, it was not what I wanted. But it was all necessary and excellently managed. The epidural provided good and timely pain relief.

Another woman's comments may go some way to explaining the apparent contradiction that epidurals contribute to women's sense of "control" while simultaneously appearing to remove it altogether:

I was not prepared for the pain of the contractions and prior to having my epidural (at the midwife's suggestion) I wondered how I would get through the rest of the labour. Having had the epidural I felt marvellous, so relieved to be pain free and in control and able to enjoy the labour. I must say I was frightened of having an epidural as I was afraid of paralysis from something going wrong. The anaesthetist, however, relieved all my fears by patient and sympathetic and unpressuring explanation. Consequently, I consented happily to it, having previously decided totally against it.

However, when an epidural did not work, was requested but not received, or was not administered at the appropriate time with this kind of support, the woman's perception of her labour could be quite different. Here, the first woman explains these feelings quite explicitly, both in terms of her loss of control and loss of faith in those attending her, while the second is again persuaded, against her own judgement, to submit to a drug she knows will not be helpful:

The epidural I had was given too late, long after I had asked for it, and due to this delay I felt that I lost control . . . also it didn't remove all the pain as I was led to expect, and the second stage was very painful.

At 8pm I asked for an epidural. I was told that no doctor was available. At 9.30 I was in agony, still no doctor was available and would I like some pethidine, which I did not want, but was given. At 10.00 I was very cross and insisted I wanted an epidural only to be told it was far too late, the baby would be born soon. I had a very painful labour, and felt very dizzy and faint afterward caused by pethidine which I did not want. On my records it did state NO pethidine. I do feel if I was given an epidural, I would of had a good labour.

Worse still, having to endure the ministrations of an inept or unsympathetic anaesthetist can reduce the entire birthing process to a nightmarish Kafkaesque experience, as this woman discovered:

> I asked for an epidural when I was 8 weeks pregnant. On the day of the birth the anaesthetist said he would prefer to do a spinal block which would be the same as the epidural. After 45 minutes of him prodding and me screaming he decided he could not use this method as I have a "bony spine". He then said we will have to give you a general anaesthetic. I said, no I want an epidural. He finally agreed to go ahead. It took about 10 minutes to insert and worked brilliantly. Why could he not do the epidural straight away? Answer – spinal block is quicker!

It is certainly interesting to note here that the anaesthetist's expediency and lack of skill was couched in terms of the woman's alleged (and hardly uncommon) inadequacy in having a "bony spine"!

Often, the problem with epidurals was related to the need for "top-ups", and the difficulties that arose from this. The anaesthesia could wear off just when they needed it most, as happened here:

> I opted for an epidural. This was inserted within half an hour and gave me total pain relief. My only regret was, having become fully dilated, I refused a top-up. I wanted to feel the urge to push and feel the sensation of giving birth. It was a great shock going from being completely pain-free to excruciating pain. Fortunately this only lasted one hour and I was greatly helped through this by my caring and supportive midwife.

Alternatively, the top-up was sometimes given too late, as in this case:

> An epidural was given quite near the start of true labour as I was in pain. It was very effective. However, I needed a top-up quite near the end (although at the time it didn't look as if I was nearing the end). This top-up resulted in my having no feeling whatsoever when trying to push and resulted in forceps being necessary.

In some hospitals, though not all, midwives are not allowed the responsibility of giving "top-ups", and it is this inter-professional power division, combined with the limited availability of anaesthetists, that contributes to delays in administering such pain relief. Indeed, staffing difficulties and non-availability were frequently mentioned by the study health professionals as reasons for epidurals not being given when requested. Women were also aware of these staffing problems, and often expressed their unhappiness about the situation with varying degrees of understanding. One woman, for example, queried whether cost was a consideration when deciding whether or not an epidural would be given:

> I have had four children now and on each occasion I was never offered epidural as a form of pain relief in labour. I feel that this form of pain relief is positively discouraged, perhaps because of the cost? Or is it because of the inconvenience of having to employ an anaesthetist?

As some of the previous quotes suggest, the use of pethidine was particularly revealing in the context of the medicalization of childbirth as a means of subordinating and controlling women. There was considerable disagreement between delivery suite professionals and women about the value of pethidine as an anaesthetic, and frequent instances of women's resistance to its use. Here the language used to describe its employment and effect included images of coercion. Several women complained about the sometimes cavalier manner with which it was administered, as though it were a means of obtaining a submissive patient rather than a pain-free labour for the woman:

> Pethidine at its height was one of the most frightening experiences I have ever had, rendering me unable to communicate with the staff or my husband. I was in a state of semi-awareness, but fully aware of the pain. Had I not had the pethidine, I would have been able to explain to the midwife that I was already in the second stage of labour when the epidural was given.

> I felt that the painkillers were forced on me rather, but the midwives knew I had a strong and violent birth and only did it in my best interest, although I find pethidine makes you out of control, but with such strong pain there was not a lot else available. I had thrombosis last year so the epidural was out.

> I felt forced to accept pethidine, even though I had categorically stated that I didn't want it.

Such comments are not only critical of the management of childbirth, they also imply that the woman's own previous experience of childbirth is not acknowledged as relevant. It is this very experience that, at the same time as enabling them to know what to expect of labour, also reminds them that the staff are failing them in some way.

"Alternative" methods of pain relief

Attitudes towards one fairly recent innovation, the use of TENS, high-lighted the ambivalence of both staff and women towards "alternative" methods of pain relief. On the one hand, TENS is a technological device provided by the hospital and thus sanctioned by doctors; on the other hand, it is perceived and used by women as an alternative to drugs. TENS is completely within the woman's control in the sense that she operates it when needed. However, its availability is controlled by the hospital. This was a source of considerable contention. Professionals seemed less convinced of its therapeutic value, which may partly explain its limited availability. It is perhaps significant in the context of women regaining control over their labour for themselves that private rental services have begun to operate in some hospitals, enabling women who can afford it to control availability as well as use. The difficulty women often had in obtaining the equipment, persuading staff to let them try it, or learning about the method in the first place, was a common source of complaint:

> Having used TENS during the labour and delivery of my second child with a good deal of success coping with pain, I was very keen to repeat this method. However, on inquiring at my GP antenatal classes, I found that availability of TENS was very limited to one in the labour ward, and one with physiotherapists, which they would lend if not in use. As my labour started quite slowly, I was able to organize from home by phone to have TENS located and left ready for my arrival. It was fortunate that no-one else had the only two sets in use! I feel it would be helpful if more of these sets were available, and am sure many mothers would appreciate the opportunity to sample this pain control method.

> Pain relief was not discussed during antenatal visits. As I went into labour, the midwife asked me what I wanted, but it was already too late for pethidine, which I thought I might need. Luckily, labour was quick and not too painful, but I would have liked to have found out about TENS.

One alternative method of pain relief that would not have been considered if the women's comments had not been taken into account, was that of nipple stimulation. This woman's surreptitious use of the method discloses a subtle subversion of the midwife's perceived power over the labour process:

> This technique is one I certainly wish I'd known about earlier, and probably contributed more than anything to a most rewarding

and enjoyable experience. My husband was pleased to be able to contribute more than just watching and feeling helpless as I endured a long, painful labour . . . I was able to reduce my labour time vastly and avoid drips entirely; consequently, I felt better and was able to cope with the pain and feel more in control of the experience. I was dubious about nipple stimulation, initially, thinking it would be embarrassing, but my husband held my hand over my chest and just gently rubbed my nipple with his thumb over the gown, and this was all it took. I don't think any of the midwives present were aware, so my worries were unfounded and we were both thrilled by its success. I still needed some pain relief but for a much shorter time.

Similarly, another woman, who had been actively able to choose her own way of giving birth and the support she needed, advocated this arrangement with great enthusiasm and showed a very positive attitude towards the pain involved:

I had a home birth with the independent midwives, without pain relief, because I believe pain is a part of childbirth. The forms of pain relief I used were being able to move around, yelling, massage, a bath, and being at home in my own environment where I felt relaxed and calm.

As these quotes suggest, it is in contexts such as these that, "other resources" including social support come into play and have a crucial bearing upon the "success" or "failure" not only of the birth process, but the subjective sense of "satisfaction" or "dissatisfaction" that ensues. Hence it is to this particular issue that the chapter now turns.

Social support in labour management

Social support in pregnancy and labour has received considerable attention in recent years (Oakley et al. 1990, Oakley 1992), and there was a great deal of evidence of its value, and of the damage caused by its absence, in this study. In particular, women often found their midwives' practical support with breathing and relaxation exercises very helpful, as in this woman's case:

I think that my birth was helped more by the midwife making me concentrate on my breathing. She was very helpful so I didn't need the gas and air until near the end of the labour.

However, such help wasn't always forthcoming or appropriate. Even women who have attended relaxation classes may find that the reality of labour makes the techniques learnt difficult to apply in practice, and at least one woman felt she would have managed better with more support during labour:

> My pain would have been better controlled had my midwife been more conversant with pain relief techniques other than drugs. I would have found support in breathing, etc., very helpful.

It was obvious from the women's responses that where they felt the professional attending them seemed to understand what they were going through and provided appropriate analgesia and encouragement, then the support and relief they were given helped enormously, even if it meant that they had a different kind of labour from the one they had anticipated or planned. The dynamics of this relationship seem to be that where support is given, confidence is engendered, and the sense of control over the labour is retained by the woman. However, there may be times during labour when the pain is so severe that women cannot help but lose that control. If these phases occur in the context of support from midwives and doctors, who know when to intervene and when to step back, then there develops a relationship that is both deferential and dialectic. Social support of this nature enabled women to take control of their labour, enhanced their self-esteem and thus, by altering their perception of the pain they were inevitably enduring, made it more bearable.

Sometimes, however, professionals did not listen to the woman's assessment of either the stage she had achieved or the extent of her pain. Indeed, the quantitative secondary analysis of the study data (Rajan 1993) showed that between 6 and 7 per cent of all professionals judged the pain relief method used to be ineffective when the women thought it effective, while 5 per cent of both obstetricians and anaesthetists, and more than one-tenth of midwives thought the method effective when the women judged it to be unsatisfactory. Moreover, the analysis showed that all professional groups were more likely to agree with each other than they were with the women. Where these situations of differing perceptions obtained, the women's suffering could be greatly and unnecessarily increased, as these comments suggest:

> Midwives don't seem to listen to the patient. They have their ideas about labour and think they know best. Each patient should be treated as an individual.

The last delivery was the most painful I experienced. I knew I was just about to deliver and on telling the midwife this she examined me and told me I wouldn't deliver for some hours yet. I said I was sure my baby was coming and was told it wasn't. My child was born less than 20 minutes later. I felt that this midwife should have trusted my judgement more than she did.

I had wanted and expected another pain-free birth but what upset me most was the fact that no-one seemed to acknowledge the level of pain that I was in or what stage of labour I had reached.

Where this inability to listen and value the woman's own contribution is combined with uncaring attitudes, she is in a particularly powerless situation. One woman, for example, had very unfortunate experiences with more than one member of staff:

During my labour of 16 hours I had care from 5 midwives and 3 doctors. One midwife was unnecessarily threatening, saying things like "You are not in enough pain" and "I'm going to really give you some pain". She then turned my drip from 5 to 40 drops a minute and insisted on giving me meptid. This treatment caused a lot of stress and upset as I became frightened of her. One doctor stood in the doorway and said, "Give her an epidural, episiotomy and forceps" then walked off. Totally impersonal, and all the things I did not want. Half an hour later I delivered with gas and air and a 2 degree tear but at least normal. This need not have occurred and certainly lowered my confidence and greatly upset both my husband and myself.

Perhaps the ultimate consequence of insensitive and unsupportive behaviour on the part of staff was expressed by one woman who eventually had a Caesarean under general anaesthetic. She was particularly upset at the large amount of invasive treatment she had received, at the ineffectiveness of all the pain relief she was given, and especially at her inability to communicate her needs to the staff in attendance:

I had an emergency Caesarean after 26 hours in labour. I had pethidine, gas and air, epidural, forceps and then Caesarean with general anaesthetic. I felt I was left too long between having an epidural and Caesarean (18 hours). I kept saying I was in too much pain and couldn't cope. No-one seemed to take any notice. I had very little say in any of the pain relief and doctors took very little notice of what I had to say. This has put me off having any more children!

Discussion

Other research has found that the use of technology and drugs to alleviate minor illnesses is viewed critically by women, whereas high technology tends to be more highly valued (Gabe & Calnan 1989). This is reflected in the realm of childbirth. Women on the whole do not want to be rendered helpless vessels from which a baby is extracted; they want to be the person who, with minimum help, pushes the baby into the world. Yet they may still allow themselves to be persuaded that by rejecting technological intervention they are putting their baby and themselves "at risk". Their responsibility for the life and safety of another individual serves to compromise them, and may cause them, in a situation where their confidence and self-esteem may be low for other reasons, to agree to procedures that they may not otherwise have considered. Moreover, the nature of pain is such that opportunities for its relief are likely to be actively sought, and, if effective, readily appreciated.

In particular, the use of TENS and Entonox clearly illustrates the contradictions inherent in women's relationship to medicalized childbirth. Women seem to be prepared to accept the benefit of medical/technological progress, including pain relief, as long as they perceive themselves to have control over its use, or see the technology as control-enhancing or restoring. Delivery room professionals (or those who administer the funding) may choose to provide these methods or not, thereby retaining ultimate control themselves. As far as TENS is concerned, women who can afford to are now able to rent their own device for the duration of labour. Evidence of this nature suggests that, though women may indeed be victims of the medicalization process in many ways, they are not always passive, as some of their comments have illustrated. Indeed, as Evans (1985) argues, women's contradictory attitudes towards medical technology need to be seen as the product of the historical struggles over childbirth in which the male obstetrician rose to ascendency, and the confused representations of pregnancy and motherhood that have resulted from these changes. In addition, she also attributes women's deference to the "doctor knows best" ideology to the asymmetry of information between doctors and patients, together with the socialized respect for professionals with specialized training, and the male sex in general (Lupton 1994: 153). This in turn supports Kohler Riessman's (1983) view that women have both gained and lost in the process of medicalization, and are not simply passive victims. In this sense, the "control stripping" nature of pain is remedied, but the price to pay may be a loss of autonomy.

As we have seen, differing perceptions of pain relief may give rise to limited responses to women's pain on the part of delivery room professionals. For instance, midwives may not give sufficient recognition to the importance of breathing and relaxation as contributing to the woman's sense of control over her pain, and thus may not provide the encouragement, support and consistent advice needed for successful perseverance with these techniques. There were many instances in which perceptions of the effectiveness of anaesthesia differed widely between the women and the professionals who attended them, particularly where the woman felt that her pain was not helped by the method yet the professional believed that it was. Where this happens, the woman may experience both the physical pain and a sense of powerlessness. In such circumstances, those whom she expects to be able to relieve her pain not only fail to do so, but are under the mistaken impression that they have succeeded, and so are not sympathetic to her suffering nor motivated to try something else.

One explanation for the discrepancies between women's and other health care professionals' perceptions of the efficacy of pain relief is that the latter are comparing each woman's labour with a whole range of others they have conducted, some of which may have been very traumatic (Bradley et al. 1983). In contrast, for the woman herself, labour will be one of the most painful and significant events she has ever experienced. Thus her frame of reference is likely to be quite different. Health professionals too, may find their work less distressing if they can minimize the suffering that they believe women undergo. While this belief may have the effect of making life more comfortable for them, it may also serve, where it is mistaken, to reduce the sense of obligation to take remedial action. Because all this is unspoken, and because neither woman nor professional fully understands the reality of each other's feelings and beliefs, the problem is self-perpetuating. It may also, in some instances, be exacerbated by the communication problems caused by social and cultural differences. A major component of the issue here is the lack of communication and understanding of the woman's need for choice and involvement in decision making about her labour and proposed pain relief. Such choice can only be based on information about the level of pain to be expected, and the methods available to control it.

The divergences between women and health professionals in perceptions of how women's pain is to be alleviated is a matter for concern in itself: when it is set against the apparently larger amount of agreement over the same issues between the various professionals involved, the matter becomes even more disturbing. These findings suggest that not only do women believe that the full extent of their pain is seldom recognized, but that because there is more rapport between professionals, it is their opinions and judgements that are likely to prevail when more effective methods are requested, or needed, by the women. The powerlessness engendered by the absence of support that is an inevitable consequence of this situation can only contribute to the women's loss of control over labour.

Sometimes pain relief is not judged by members of the medical staff to be in the woman's or baby's "best interest". In many cases, as long as the woman understands the reasons behind this kind of decision, and agrees with them – in other words, gives her informed consent – she maintains a sense of control over her situation, however limited, and may come to view her subsequent suffering with equanimity. However, where this informed consent is not sought, the experience may be even more distressing.

Too often, extraneous factors are allowed to influence the process and interfere with the arrival of pain relief. Clearly, requests for epidurals that are met with delay caused by the non-availability of anaesthetists result in considerable suffering, as does the withholding of other drugs because the only person qualified to give them is busy elsewhere. While such occurrences may not derive directly from the subordination of the labouring woman, they are nevertheless consequences of a medical system whose focus is on the safeguarding of professional mystique, and whose budget priorities are not necessarily those of satisfactory patient care. As Oakley (1993: 129) remarks:

> It often seems to outsiders that an institution such as a maternity hospital exists not to provide services for mothers but to justify its own existence. One is led to the impression that many people who run hospitals feel that they would do so much more efficiently if there were no patients at all.

There were numerous occasions when delivery room professionals seemed particularly powerless to improve the women's pain control. The prevalence of such complaints as the unit being too busy, and inadequate staffing or facilities suggested widespread under-resourcing of maternity units and consequent overworking of existing staff, all of which could result in inadequate levels of pain relief being given.

Women know that pain is almost inevitable during childbirth and that no pain relief method guarantees a pain-free labour. The crucial issue is whether they perceive their pain as bearable, and that is largely dependent on their sense of control over the process. Health professionals have the means to alleviate that pain, but to do so effectively the method used has to be tailored to the needs of the individual woman, with her informed consent and her understanding of the effect and awareness of the alternatives. Furthermore, emotional support to reinforce the woman's sense of control over the situation enables her to view pain in a constructive way, to retain her self-esteem and her confidence in the help she is receiving.

Acknowledgements

The analysis of the NBTF survey data was funded by the Department of Health in 1992 and carried out at the Social Science Research Unit, part of London University's Institute of Education. The author would like to thank Professor Ann Oakley for her advice and support.

References

Arney, W. R. & J. Neill 1983. The location of pain in childbirth. *Sociology of Health and Illness* **7**, 109–17.

Bradley, C., C. R. Brewin, S. L. B. Duncan 1983. Perceptions of labour: discrepancies between midwives' and patients' ratings. *British Journal of Obstetrics and Gynaecology* **90**, 1176–9.

Cartwright, A. 1987. *The dignity of labour?* London: Tavistock.

Bendelow, G. 1992. *Gender and perceptions of pain*. PhD thesis, University of London.

Chamberlain, G., P. Steer, A. Wraight (eds) 1993. *The 1990 pain relief in labour survey*. Edinburgh: Churchill Livingstone.

Cohen, F. L. 1980. Postsurgical pain relief: patients' status and nurses' medication choices. *Pain* **9**, 265–74.

Dickersin, K. 1989. Pharmacological control of pain during labour. In *Effective care in pregnancy and childbirth*, I. Chalmers, M. Enkin, M. J. N. C. Keirse (eds), 913–50. Oxford: Oxford University Press.

Drew, N. C., P. Salmon, L. Webb 1989. Mothers', midwives' and obstetricians' views on the features of obstetric care which influence satisfaction with childbirth. *British Journal of Obstetrics and Gynaecology* **96**, 1084–8.

Evans, F. 1985. Managers and labourers: women's attitudes to reproductive technology. In *Smothered by technology: technology in women's lives*, W. Faulkner & E. Arnold (eds), 109–27. London: Pluto.

Gabe, J. & M. Calnan 1989. The limits of medicine: women's perception of medical technology. *Social Science and Medicine* **28**(3), 223–31.

Green, J., V. Coupland, J. Kitzinger 1988. *Great expectations: a prospective study of women's expectations and experiences of childbirth*. Unpublished report, Child Care and Development Group, University of Cambridge.

Johnston, M. 1976. Communication of patients' feelings in hospital. In *Communications between doctors and patients*, A. E. Bennett. London: Nuffield Provincial Hospitals Trust.

Kirke, P. N. 1980a. Mothers' views of obstetric care. *British Journal of Obstetrics and Gynaecology* **87**, 1029–33.

Kirke, P. N. 1980b. Mothers' views of care in labour. *British Journal of Obstetrics and Gynaecology*, **87** 1034–8.

Kohler Riessman, C. 1983. Women and medicalization: a new perspective. *Social Policy* **14**, 3–18.

Lupton, D. 1994. *Medicine as culture: illness, disease and the body in western societies*. London: Sage.

Marks, R. M. & E. J. Sachar 1973. Undertreatment of medical inpatients with narcotic analgesics. *Annals of Internal Medicine* **78**(2), 173–81.

McCaffery, M. & L. Hart 1976. Undertreatment of acute pain with narcotics. *American Journal of Nursing* **76**(10), 1586–91.

Melzack, R. 1990. The tragedy of needless pain. *Scientific American* **262**(2), 19–25.

Morgan, B. M., C. J. Bulpitt, P. Clifton 1982. Analgesia and satisfaction in childbirth (The Queen Charlotte's 1000 mother survey). *The Lancet*, 9 October, 808–10.

Oakley, A. 1984. *The captured womb*. Oxford: Blackwell.

Oakley, A. 1992. *Social support and motherhood*. Oxford: Blackwell.

Oakley, A. 1993. *Women, medicine and health*. Edinburgh: Edinburgh University Press.

Oakley, A., L. Rajan, A. Grant 1990. Social support and pregnancy outcome: report of a randomised controlled trial. *British Journal of Obstetrics and Gynaecology* **97**, 155–62.

Rajan, L. 1992. "Not just me dreaming": the disruption and facilitation of mourning after pregnancy loss. *Health Visitor* **65**(10), 354–7.

Rajan, L. 1993. Perceptions of pain and pain relief in labour: the gulf between experience and observation. *Midwifery* **9**, 136–45.

Rajan, L. 1994. The impact on breastfeeding of obstetric procedures and anaesthesia/analgesia during labour and delivery. *Midwifery* **10**, 87–103.

Simkin, P. 1989. Non-pharmacological methods of pain relief during labour. In *Effective care in pregnancy and childbirth*, I. Chalmers, M. Enkin, M. J. N. C. Keirse (eds). Oxford: Oxford University Press.

Stanworth, M. (ed.) 1987. *Reproductive technologies: gender, motherhood & medicine*. Cambridge: Polity.

Chapter 10

New reproductive technologies: the views of women undergoing treatment

Elaine Denny

We may never have children, but at least [we] can look at pictures of [our] embryos (Mary: IVF recipient).

The possibility of conception taking place outside the uterus became a reality in 1978 with the birth of the first child following in vitro fertilization (IVF). Since then the technology of assisted reproduction has developed to include modifications of the IVF technique, and recently the birth of babies to post-menopausal women. The continuing development of these procedures has provoked strong emotions, both from those who wish to see them used with few restrictions, and from those who oppose their continued use (Stacey 1992). The most vociferous have tended to be scientists and the medical profession, who see assisted reproduction as medical progress, and feminists, especially radical feminists (although many cannot be easily compartmentalized), who perceive it as a continuation of the male monopoly of reproduction. Hidden from the debate has been the perspective of women who decide to undergo these therapies as treatment for infertility.

One of the main themes of radical feminism is the question of who has power and control over reproduction. IVF is perceived as part of the male attempt to control female sexuality and fertility, and needs to be placed in this context. Although IVF is promoted as a treatment for infertility, the emphasis on technology is about control of reproductive capacity.

The justification for the development of procedures such as IVF has always been to "help" infertile couples to conceive, to offer them a choice, but Spallone (1989) and Crowe (1990) argue that this is not the case, that IVF is not about fertility particularly and can never be a treatment for fertility problems. They call IVF a "technological fix" for the social condition of childlessness, one that bypasses the causes of infertility and starts with the viewpoint of infertility as being a "medical problem".

Stanworth (1987) states that women are blinded by science and manipulated into accepting new technologies – a technological imperative. Male doctors use women's intense desire for children to manipulate them into experimentation, and support of any procedure that produces them (Rowland 1987a). Women's desire for children is therefore fuelled by pronatalist ideologies, and exploited by men who use technology to turn their illusions of reproductive power into a reality (Stanworth 1987). While radical feminist research has tended, with a few exceptions (e.g. Crowe 1985, Klein 1989), to seek a theoretical understanding of reproductive technology as a product of patriarchy with little attention to women's lived experience of infertility treatment, empirical research in contrast is often atheoretical and located in a biomedical paradigm. Consequently, both approaches tend to obscure, and therefore to invalidate, the perspective of women's own emotions and understanding of treatment (Denny 1994). Drawing upon qualitative data obtained by ten semi-focused interviews with women who were undergoing, or had recently undergone, infertility treatment by IVF or gamete intra fallopian transfer (GIFT), this chapter seeks to address and explore these issues. The interviews were based upon Graham's "surveying through stories" technique (1984: 104). She suggests that while exploitation and misrepresentation may be impossible to eliminate from social research, it is possible to minimize them by using the interview structure to encourage active participation by the respondent.

Cannon (1989) used this approach to interview women who were undergoing treatment for breast cancer:

> I decided to use semi-focused interviews using a conversational approach which allowed women to discuss a given topic in whichever way they chose . . . Although the wider structure of the interview is set by the researcher, the respondent has scope within this to construct the data, since she can choose what and how much to say on a given topic (Cannon 1989: 64).

The use of this method is problematic in that it is difficult to meet the criterion of external validity, but Graham argues that this is balanced by safeguarding the rights of informants. The fusing of data and interpretation through the story, however, means that a high degree of internal validity is achieved. Because of limited availability of IVF within the national health service (NHS) the women in the study were all attending clinics within the private sector.

Women's experience of IVF

Studies of people's experiences of modern medicine and medical care have mainly consisted of consumer satisfaction surveys. As Calnan (1988) has noted these tend to show that patients are rarely critical of medical practice, although research using other methods tends not to bear this out. Most women accept that success rates for individual IVF clinics are between 5 and 15 per cent, yet usually feel that they will be successful (Holmes & Tymstra 1987) and do not blame clinic staff when they are not. They also accept intensive drug regimes and invasive procedures, seemingly without question. Similarly, the women in the research under discussion approached IVF with a mixture of excitement and trepidation. Many of them had tried other treatments first, and IVF was a last resort. One woman, for example, described going to faith healers and acupuncturists, before deciding on IVF. It is to these experiences that I now turn.

The development of the ova and embryo transfer

For a woman the typical regime for an IVF cycle is physically very demanding, whereas the emotional demands are felt by both the man and the woman, although not always equally. Treatment begins on day one of the menstrual cycle with three-hourly nasal sprays of Buserilin, which suppresses the natural cycle, and this continues until ovulation occurs. Prednisilone tablets are taken from days 1 to 21 of the cycle in order to sensitize ovarian tissue to the effects of hormones. Injections of human menopausal gonadotrophin (Pergonal) stimulate the ovaries to produce multiple eggs and are given from day 4 until the ovarian follicles are ripe (usually around day 13). Human chorionic gonadotrophin (Profasi) is given by injection at this point to prepare the eggs for collection 35 hours later. Blood tests and ultrasound scans monitor the developing eggs in order to determine their maturity. Egg retrieval occurs under either local or general anaesthetic. Eggs are mixed with sperm and either put into the fimbral end of the fallopian tube for GIFT, or a maximum of three may be inserted into the uterus of the woman when they have been fertilized in a petri dish and reached the four cell stage (IVF). Two weeks later further blood tests can determine whether hormone levels are rising, which may indicate that a pregnancy has occurred.

The present research, in common with other studies (e.g. Sandelowski 1990), found that investigations and treatments took over people's lives. The first two weeks of the procedure in particular entails a lot of commitment for the woman going to the hospital for tests, having injections and waking three hourly during the night for the nasal spray. Mary described the first two weeks as follows:

In some ways it's kind of exalting and in some ways you're a victim. The experience itself is stressful, everyone will tell you that. The man has to make an effort but the woman is giving up everything, like drink. You go to a party and your husband gets drunk in a corner and you say "you bastard, you know you're not supposed to get drunk – it will affect the sperm".

Others commented on how they planned holidays and other events round IVF attempts, or conversely how they were determined to fit them into normal work patterns, and to give the injections themselves in an attempt not to let the treatment dominate their lives.

Interrupted sleep, daily injections and the massive build up of hormones affected all the women in the study in some way.

It's a very hard procedure to go through, very intense. You've got to live the treatment for that month. You can't get away from it . . . When I was half way through we did go to Paris for the weekend, and I took the injections with me . . . My legs were getting sore and I found just walking difficult, and I was tired because I wasn't sleeping (Sue).

The drug regime resulted in side-effects for most of the women in terms of mood swings and even hyperstimulation of the ovaries, when too many eggs mature too quickly, but these were accepted as inevitable. As Debbie commented "I felt I got through it because I knew how much I needed those eggs." By the end of the first two weeks, just before the eggs were collected, women described the effects of high levels of hormones in ways such as the following:

You're like a bitch at the end because you're so full of progesterone, your period's coming on, you've got pre-menstrual tension, the progesterone is holding your period back and your hormones are all over the place. You want to kill each other (Mary).

Some women did think about long-term effects of large doses of hormones, but only after they had discontinued treatment. For example, Jean commented: "At the time it did not even cross my mind, you just look towards the end goal." Others, however, referred to themselves as guinea pigs, and recognized the experimental nature of the treatment, but again accepted any potential risk as worthwhile if it resulted in a pregnancy. In this sense, acceptance of the procedures seemed to be rooted not in any "blind faith" in medical expertise, but simply as a means to an end. As most couples had endured years of investigations and procedures they viewed remaining childless as being their only alternative to IVF. However, it is also true that these women, like those in the studies by Holmes & Tymstra (1987) and Milne (1988) tended to overestimate their individual chances of success. For example Anne stated "We were told quite bluntly what the statistics are. I almost had a sense of false security because everything seemed to go so well." This may be necessary in order to rationalize the investment of time, pain and money that IVF involves. Despite many setbacks most women had great hope and faith in their own ultimate success.

The procedure for egg collection and fertilization was viewed with a mixture of apprehension and excitement.

> I was terrified of the aspiration [to remove the eggs from the ovary] but they said I was one of the stillest they had, because I can remember lying there clenching my fist thinking how desperately I needed those eggs (Debbie).

GIFT is a one-stage procedure, therefore until a pregnancy is confirmed or menstruation begins it is not known how the procedure is progressing. With IVF, egg retrieval is followed by a 48 hour wait to find out whether fertilization has taken place. This can be a time of great competition. Mary commented "We've achieved three embryos each time and it's a kind of upmanship. How many embryos did you get? It is very competitive." There is a feeling of success knowing that eggs have fertilized, although this can be short lived. One couple's experience is typical.

> There were tears when we found out, they phoned and said "Can you come, we've got three embryos." After they're put back you sit there knowing there's three embryos inside you. . . . You honestly believe you are pregnant. I know it's silly. I knew they had to embed. I felt one had to "take" at least. You don't imagine it not working (Anne).

Franklyn (1992) notes how definitions of "success" change with unsuccessful IVF attempts. To begin with the criterion of success is what is often labelled the "take home baby", but as this continues to be elusive the concept of success becomes redefined, so that fertilized embryos, or chemical pregnancy (i.e. a rise in hormone levels consistent with a pregnancy occurring, which subsequently proves not to have happened) is regarded as "success". As Mary put it "We are assured of slight success by the fact that we can produce embryos."

The second two weeks of the cycle

The following two weeks, waiting to know whether a pregnancy had occurred was a very stressful time for all the women in the study. Along with the uncertainty some felt a great responsibility for the fate of the embryos:

> The aspiration, I was frightened of it and it hurt, but that's only one day. The two weeks of waiting for the result, waiting for the blood test, that's hard the whole time (Debbie).

The women who saw each hurdle as success, and who perceived themselves as having a good chance of conceiving were more likely to feel excitement along with anxiety. They typically described themselves as pleased and increasingly confident as each hurdle was surmounted, especially if they had actually seen the fertilized embryos prior to embryo transfer.

Franklyn suggests that for couples receiving IVF, the apparently "simple" act of conception is broken down into stages, all of which are technologically complex and subject to the "clinical and scientific gaze" (1992: 83). Each stage becomes highly visible, and ultimate failure is then unexpected and extremely disappointing. As John put it:

> You're so ecstatic one minute with joy that everything's going so well. You think you've done it . . . You go from the very heights to the bottom with just one phone call.

His wife described her third unsuccessful attempt of assisted reproduction, the previous two having been GIFT:

> It was worse with IVF, knowing that you'd had three eggs put back. It doesn't hit you straight away. No one who hasn't been through this can understand what it feels like. We've both lost people close to us, but this is a different type of grieving, you have got nothing to remember what you are grieving for and it is devastating.

Along with grief some women experienced guilt when a pregnancy did not occur. Women wondered whether, by their actions or behaviour since embryo transfer, they had done something to prevent the embryos implanting, or even subconsciously rejected them. As Mary said "You feel responsible for rejecting those embryos."

Two women in the study had become pregnant by GIFT (one gave birth to triplets, but one of the babies died shortly after birth, the other had one child), and one had conceived naturally. None of these women wanted to have IVF or GIFT again, as they found it quite traumatic. As one woman who has since suffered panic attacks and agoraphobia stated:

> People say I seemed to sail through it at the time because I knew I had to, and all the way through the five years I had to keep myself thinking positive and keep going through everything . . . Yet for the past two years I've suffered from panic attacks. It has been suggested that it's the stress of the past five years coming out now (Debbie).

Only two of the women without children decided not to continue in an IVF programme, one following hyperstimulation of ovaries with a subsequent miscarriage, the other being a woman who only ever wanted two attempts.

The rest of the sample were determined to continue as long as possible, until they were considered too old by the clinic. For example, Anne commented: "I'll go on as long as I can until I'm 42, which is how old they are doing it to, but after that – I'm dreading the day. I don't know how I'll cope with that.

To summarize, the women in this study were, on the whole, very positive about their inclusion in an IVF programme despite the fact that the treatment, to a large extent, took over their lives. Although the procedure is physically stressful the majority of women felt that the ends justified the means, and that the chance of having a baby, albeit a small one, was worth the financial, emotional and in some cases physical cost. The definition of "success", therefore, became redefined as IVF proved unsuccessful for most women, and the chance of individual success by any definition tended to be overestimated. These strategies probably helped to rationalize continuation in a programme, the cost of which is high and the outcome extremely uncertain.

What then, do these accounts tell us about the relevance, or otherwise, of feminist perspectives on the new reproductive technologies? The following sections will concentrate on using these experiences and other data to explore the radical feminist position in relation to IVF. Radical feminism is, undoubtedly, a broad church, but for the purposes of this chapter there is a common emphasis on the control of women's reproductive role by men as the root of patriarchal oppression; the oldest and most widespread form of oppression.

Pronatalism and IVF

The ideology of pronatalism is of major importance for radical feminists in explaining why women "collude" in practices that are not ultimately in their interests. Even though the chances of becoming pregnant through IVF are small, many women are prepared to undergo the physical and emotional stress described in the previous section in order to achieve parenthood by this method. This fact is often used to further justify the technique, as Rowland argues "essentially and misleadingly in the catch-cry that 'women want it'" (1985: 541). She goes on to argue that in a pronatalist culture women only want it because their identity as adult females depends on it. Women are accorded status through their reproductive capacity, in order to be fulfilled they must reproduce. People marry with the expectation that they will reproduce, they parent because it brings social approval and because all social structures deem parenting and family life to be good (Rowland 1984a).

The implementation of IVF programmes, with their emphasis on conception and the production of offspring, together with their neglect of other forms of parenting, is seen to reinforce a biological notion of motherhood, with the result that the social meaning of motherhood and maternal instinct is lost (Crowe 1990). Yet this approach, by portraying women purely as a social group, and the infertile as victims of the ideology of motherhood, ignores the diversity of experience among individuals. For example, Warren (1988) argues that many women on IVF programmes are actually well informed, both about the nature of the treatment and the social construction of motherhood, and that reproductive autonomy must include the right to take risks with our own bodies.

None of the women in the present study introduced the subject of pronatalism spontaneously, although some did make reference to it. For example Mary, while addressing her own upbringing, said "the whole thing is very primitive, you get down to very primitive instincts. Man goes out and gets meat, woman stays home and has children." Most of the women found that infertility affected their self-esteem, not just in terms of childbearing but in all aspects of their lives. Even where women were highly confident and independent before knowing of their infertility, on discovery their self-esteem was severely affected. Some women spoke of not feeling a "complete woman", while others spoke of being outsiders within their social circle.

Not all women, however, perceived themselves this way. Some women saw their childlessness as an opportunity to achieve in other areas of life, especially professional women who had received promotions. While some women saw pronatalist pressures as influencing their decision to undertake IVF, others felt it was something they did for themselves. Many of these described a baby as "icing on the cake" or a bonus, something they very much wanted, but not something that was essential to their lives. It would seem that infertile couples, far from entering IVF programmes blindly, actually spend a great deal of time evaluating their decisions. One woman described how she and her husband re-examined their feelings before every course of treatment to decide if it was still what they both wanted. Another commented "At least with IVF it's a conscious decision, whereas with the other way it's not conscious – you can get drunk and it happens in the back of a car." During the Gulf War she had seriously considered whether she wanted children. Women, then, have diverse views on the ideology of pronatalism, and the extent to which it influences decision making. The next section will encompass these issues in a broader discussion of power and control in reproductive technology.

Power and control over reproductive technology

Obviously issues concerning the power of the medical profession and technological imperatives are not confined to problems of fertility, but infertility is somewhat different to other areas of medical interest. It would appear on the surface that infertile women have more control than other patients. Infertility is something for which a couple may or may not choose medical intervention. In this respect most couples in the present study consulted their general practitioner (GP) only after one or two years of unprotected intercourse, although some were not referred to a specialist immediately. As with other areas of health care, GPs act as gatekeepers for specialist services, and it was at this level that some couples found opposition to their wishes. For example, one woman was told to go away and adopt a child.

Having been accepted for IVF treatment the woman has to initiate each treatment cycle, she must make contact with the clinic in order for treatment to begin. Women spoke of delaying treatment until they felt mentally prepared, or of taking temporary breaks in treatment. One woman refused to have IVF, because she did not have confidence in the clinic she was attending, and so transferred to another one in order to begin IVF.

Although most women were not given a choice between different technologies (e.g. between IVF and GIFT), the rationale for the treatments was usually explained to them and accepted. Counselling was invariably given before treatment commenced, but by that point many women had already made the decision to have IVF. Having had one form of treatment unsuccessfully, some women requested another and received it. One woman requested IVF after two attempts with GIFT, another wanted IVF following unsuccessful artificial insemination.

None of the women felt that being in an IVF programme meant their lives were being manipulated by doctors or medical science, although some did express feelings of vulnerability and a reliance on doctors to retrieve and implant the eggs. Indeed more women actually felt that IVF gave them back control, as infertility meant a loss of control. As Mary put it "your body is letting you down". Whereas radical feminists describe infertile women as passively accepting the control of a male medical profession, women themselves view acceptance of infertility as passive, and making decisions and using the technology as regaining control (Denny 1994).

Other empirical research has also found that infertility, rather than medical technology, gives women a sense of powerlessness. In Milne's study, for example, the most common coping mechanism adopted was "vigilant focusing" (1988: 351), an active seeking of information and compulsive attention to details of investigation and treatment. Franklyn too suggests that couples acquire a vast amount of information about the process of fertilization and implantation, but although knowledge does not give them the power to affect their situation it does give them a sense of control. Strickler (1992) found control to be a recurring theme within the literature, with couples feeling that they are exerting control over their lives by pursuing all options, rather than passively accepting their fate. This perspective would appear to contradict that of feminist writers concerning women's experience of medical technology. In reviewing this literature Gabe & Calnan found that the image presented "would seem to be one of women being prevented from taking control of their health as a result of medical technology"(1989: 224). They suggest that a view of professional dominance and patient subordination is too simplistic at the level of doctor–patient interaction, which needs to be seen in terms of co-operation as well as power.

Choice and reproductive technology

In choosing to use technology women may, as Klein (1987) states, be basing that choice on information that is one sided and male centred, but Rothman argues that choices are very rarely totally free.

> Perhaps what we should realise is that human beings living in society have very little choice ever. There may be no such thing as individual choice in a social structure, not in any absolute way. The social structure creates needs, the need for perfect children – and creates the technology which enables people to make the needed choices. The question is not whether choices are con-

structed but *how* they are constructed (Rothman 1984: 32, original emphasis).

The issue of how choices are constructed has been crucial in determining whether women are manipulated, or whether they are fully aware of the constraints that influence their decision making. In choosing NRTs women have been accused of being "blinded by science"(Stanworth 1987), brainwashed by pronatalist ideologies (Hanmer 1987) and not given adequate information (Klein 1987), which renders them incapable of making a "reasoned choice". Birke (1990), on the other hand, argues that although all choices made by men or women take place within a social and material context, people are capable of recognizing this and taking it into account.

Certainly, the women in this research felt that they had a right to exercise reproductive choice in deciding to use every means available in order to have a child. Lupton argues that it should be a woman's right to choose how they use or reject reproductive technology, and that "feminism has largely failed to recognise the possibility of using medical technology as a resource" (Lupton 1994: 159).

When certain choices are available, they may become the socially endorsed alternative, and other choices may be lost or become less acceptable as a consequence. One of the other options for childless couples is, of course, that of adoption, which would fulfil the social, if not the biological need for a child. Eight women considered adoption, but adoption agencies in the UK will only consider couples who have discontinued or rejected fertility treatment and many have age limits, so that couples are forced to go in one direction or the other. Their choices are curtailed, not by the medical profession, but by other parts of the social structure. Women were more likely than their husbands to want to adopt a child, and this is borne out by other studies (e.g. Crowe 1985). However, they were unwilling to terminate all fertility treatment in order to do so. Most women felt that having a child was more important than actually conceiving and giving birth to it, and the majority of men concurred. Crowe interpreted her findings as evidence that men define their relationship with a child purely in biological terms, while women considered the social relationship. IVF, she argued, was reinforcing a male-centred view of parenthood, by reinforcing conception.

The experience of medical practice

Although none of the women perceived themselves to be controlled by the medical profession, most were aware of financial constraints on themselves and others. Availability of IVF on the National Health Service is limited, and many purchasers of health care are opting out of fertility treatment. Consequently, the number of IVF attempts and the interval between them was a mainly financial decision. Many women had to save to pay for each attempt within the private health care sector. One woman even borrowed money using her house as security in order to finance two attempts at IVF. Certainly these women were very aware that for many IVF was not an option because of financial constraints, and expressed the opinion that fertility treatment should be more widely available within the health service.

However, despite financial constraints, women felt that they had control over their treatment, because they could go elsewhere if dissatisfied, although this did involve returning to their GP as gatekeeper. One woman, for example, refused to have IVF at a particular clinic because she did not have confidence in the staff:

> We didn't see the same nurses or doctor twice and there was just a great big waiting room full of people, no one had any time for you and you really did get the feeling that they just wanted the money (Debbie).

Mary also changed clinics due to dissatisfaction with the way she was treated:

> This 28 year old houseman said "You're a mess aren't you" and I've never thought of myself as a mess before, and it's labelling you as "infertile" and a "mess".

Strickler (1992) states that, with few exceptions, medical literature on reproduction and infertility is limited to the biological aspects of reproduction, and medical interventions to relieve or circumvent the causes of infertility. The social and emotional meaning of infertility for individual couples is therefore ignored. Rowland (1987b) also notes how IVF teams cope with failures in the programme by avoiding follow-up contact with those women who fail to conceive, which may explain the impersonal nature of some clinics. However, paying for treatment gave the women in this study the confidence to go elsewhere when this occurred and GPs were more willing to re-refer them than would probably be the case with NHS patients.

Other research (e.g. Crowe 1990) suggests that women are under pressure not to show signs of emotional distress and, therefore, to accept failure stoically. However, none of the women in the present study found this to be the case. Indeed, one described how she rang the clinic in tears every day for two weeks when she had a threatened miscarriage following GIFT, whereas others said they felt like individuals and "not just a file". Some couples did, however, feel that their own perceptions of what may be relevant factors in their personal situation were dismissed by doctors. For example, Anne commented:

> I've had this pain for 20 years now and had tests and they've said we can't find anything wrong with you at all, virtually it's all in your head. Now that they've found it's endometriosis all we went through [in terms of fertility treatment] was a waste of time.

Her husband added:

> [My wife] has had this pain for so long that we couldn't have any sort of regular sex life in order to try for a baby, but you can't get that through to these people.

Whereas Jean also had ideas about what could be causing her infertility:

> My periods have lasted a day at the most. All along I have thought that it was something to do with it, but everyone dismissed it and said it doesn't matter how long your periods are, it's nothing to do with it.

She later became pregnant naturally following homeopathic treatment for another health problem, which among other effects lengthened her menstruation.

As Calnan (1987) suggests, certain areas of medical practice, especially those where there is a degree of uncertainty, have the greatest potential for tension between doctor and patient. Many women on IVF programmes have unexplained infertility. As such there is considerable scope for uncertainty concerning both cause and outcome. In the present study, however, there was only limited evidence of tension; something that may be due to the willingness of patients to change clinics. In addition, it may also be illustrative of social relations of medical technology as both dialectical and deferential (Gabe & Calnan 1989); a situation in which a seemingly contradictory relationship involves elements of traditional power and mutual co-operation. Indeed, couples who have experienced long-term infertility, in common with others who have long-term conditions, become experts in their own problem, and the vigilant focusing described by Milne may give people the confidence to negotiate, rather than passively accept treatments.

Radical feminist writers point to the way in which women actually aid men in the control of reproduction, colluding in the development of technology by offering ourselves as "living laboratories" for experimentation

(Rowland 1984b). While Kohler Riessman (1989) agrees that women have been involved in these developments, she nonetheless interprets the processes very differently, stating that "women actively participated in the construction of new medical definitions" (1989: 191), but with different motives than the medical profession. Although, as the first section of the chapter testifies, some of the women in this study did indeed describe themselves as guinea pigs and acknowledged the experimental nature of some treatments, they also felt participation to be an acceptable risk, and did not actually perceive any risk to themselves personally. One woman, for example, gladly accepted the need for experimentation as necessary for the development of such procedures. Similarly, none of the women gave much thought to the possible long-term drug use and superstimulation of the ovaries, except in retrospect. Rather, most women said they were willing to try anything. According to Klein (1987) there is a lack of discussion about unknown dangers of technology, and even known dangers such as ovarian cysts, hyperstimulation of ovaries and other damage is rarely mentioned unless it happens. Steinberg (1990) states that drugs are usually named and described to patients in terms of their desired effects, particularly the effect on the ovaries; the implication being that there are no adverse effects on other organs of the body.

However, very little research has been conducted into the long-term effects of hormonal drugs, and that what has been done has focused on the effects to the foetus and resulting child, rather than the women who take them. Certainly women in the present study tended to accept even quite serious side-effects. Sarah, for example, described her hyperstimulation and subsequent septicaemia and miscarriage as just "bad luck". Indeed, she even considered continuing in the IVF programme following this, and accepted the risk philosophically stating:

> I was really very poorly, I wouldn't want to go through that again. I'd never heard of hyperstimulation until I actually got it, no one said there was any risk like that . . . I still considered having another go, because they changed the regime (Sarah).

By contrast, another woman who hyperstimulated described herself as unaffected by the drugs, and did not worry as she felt she was "well looked after" (Diane).

Some of the women had more eggs fertilized than were actually replaced, which is a common occurrence with superovulation, but none had given much thought to what happened to these other embryos. Two women had given permission for embryos not replaced to be observed for two weeks (which is the legal limit for research on embryos), but thought that after that time they would probably not survive. Whereas neither of these women thought that any experimentation would be conducted on their embryos, or that they would be used for other purposes without their permission, they were not against early experimentation on embryos.

The history of the relationship between women, their bodies and obstetrics and gynaecology is reported by Rowland to be one of "mistreatment, manipulation and mutilation" (1985: 544). Certain forms of contraception, intervention in childbirth and reproductive technology have all worked to the detriment of women. Corea et al. (1987) add that women have colluded because they have been convinced by the nature of the information given to them, that men and technology are more reliable and superior than their own bodies and experiences. Patriarchy's norms become *the* norms. As a consequence, as Burfoot (1990) argues, increased technological intervention in reproduction becomes "normalized" and innovative techniques are no longer perceived as experimental, but instead are accepted as "routine" procedures. From this perspective women are seen as having no part in the production of technology, which remains firmly in the hands of the male scientific and medical communities. Yet they are its main recipients. Knowledge remains in male hands and women can easily be persuaded to accept technical procedures, simply because they do not have the knowledge to question or challenge them.

However, to see women as universally passive in this way is to perpetuate stereotypical myths about women's actions. Indeed, as Kohler Riessman (1989) argues, this approach perpetuates assumptions about women that feminists have been trying to challenge. As we have seen, the way in which control and co-operation are experienced by women themselves is far too complex for such simplistic analyses. Certainly at the point of delivery women would appear to have control over their treatment. They define themselves as "infertile", albeit in a society that expects marriage to lead to reproduction, and they decide on medical solutions to their infertility. They initiate treatment, they withdraw either temporarily or permanently and they move from one clinic to another if dissatisfied. More subtle forms of control do, however, exist. A pronatalist culture and a powerful male-dominated medical profession that defines childlessness in medical terms encourages women to accept the emotional and physical stress of treatment and to knowingly accept inadequate information regarding drug regimes and potential side-effects. Despite this, the emphasis placed by many feminist writers on technological determinism does, however, detract from the wider issue of medical abuse, which has at its roots not only gender discrimination, but discrimination on the basis of race, class and ability. The problem with this approach, and the reason it cannot explain the relationship between control and co-operation, is the tendency to express the issues in dichotomies – medical versus lay, informed versus ignorant (Stacey 1992), ignoring the complex relationships involved.

Feminism and IVF

The research discussed in this chapter has considered the actual experience of women undergoing IVF, but it has also adopted a critical stance towards certain feminist literature bearing on this topic. In this final section I wish to develop this critique further and also to develop an alternative feminist perspective, one that legitimizes women's own experiences. The experience of individual women who have chosen IVF as a means of dealing with infertility has been missing from most radical feminist literature. Women have been portrayed as powerless victims, passively accepting whatever a male-dominated medical profession offers them. What is not addressed by radical feminism is the possibility that women may not agree with these understandings of the way larger social structures influence their everyday world. There is an implicit assumption among many feminist writers that once women have knowledge they will become self-emancipating. In contrast, as Stanley & Wise (1990) point out, oppression is a very complex process, one in which most women are rarely totally powerless. Indeed, women have often challenged male domination in reproductive issues, a recent example being the reversal in the number of induced births (Hillier 1991).

The experiences described in this chapter have been recounted by women who are undergoing, or have recently undergone, IVF. The fact that they were self-selecting, and that they had the financial means to choose reproductive technology, may have resulted in a sample of women with an exceptional sense of control over their lives, which in turn could affect the way in which they perceive patriarchal control. Self-selection may also have produced a particularly articulate and reflective group of women, who were more inclined to rationalize their position. To really examine the relevance of a radical feminist perspective effectively, therefore, a wider sample of women needs to be studied. In particular those who have been excluded from participating in IVF programmes may feel disempowered, and may conceptualize their relationship to a patriarchal social structure more critically.

As Stanley & Wise argue: "the experience of women is ontologically fractured and complex because we do not all share one single and unseamed reality" (1990: 22). Certainly, the experiences of the women in this particular study are very diverse, even though they were ostensibly undergoing the same procedure. In this respect the extent to which they conform to pronatalism, or display elements of what might be explained by radical feminists as "false consciousness" varies considerably. Yet the radical feminist tendency to treat women as a homogeneous group, universally oppressed and passive, and to treat all relationships with men as exploitative, leads to an oversimplification of what is, in fact, an extremely complex issue. As Stacey points out: "Social life is very complex" (1992: 35).

One way in which this is manifested is in the widely held assumption that the experience of women as an oppressed group has led to similarities in all women that outweigh differences of colour, class, ability and so on. Conversely, Kohler Riessman (1989) argues that although women from the dominant class used medicalization for their own needs, women from other classes only partially adopted it, at times resisting it altogether. The fertile cannot generalize from their own experiences of pronatalist ideology or power and control to include the infertile. Indeed it was often said during interviews that people with children do not understand the experience of infertility, or the motivation to participate in IVF programmes. Eisenstein calls for a "retreat from false universalism and a sensitivity to the diversity of women's needs" (1983: 141). An argument that is often used (e.g. Crowe 1990) is that new reproductive technology is not about helping women to become mothers, but about male control of reproduction. Experimentation on fertilization and on the ensuing embryos is a step in the direction of a complete take-over of reproduction using techniques such as ectogenesis, cloning and hybridization. In what Corea et al. (1987) call a "woman hating world" some feminists view this as a distinct possibility.

The reality, however, is that the newer adaptations to IVF are becoming less invasive and giving doctors less control over outcomes. GIFT allows sperm and ova to meet in the fimbral end of the fallopian tube and fertilization occurs where it would naturally. Controlled hyperstimulation and intra-uterine insemination is becoming the treatment of choice in many centres (albeit a choice made largely by professionals) for women who have patent fallopian tubes, and this requires no surgical intervention at all. On the other hand research is also currently being conducted into the possibility of removing immature ova and maturing them in vitro prior to fertilization and implantation (reducing the need for such large hormone dosages). Thus current research does not appear to be moving in any one direction, but is diverse with many objectives. It is not the technology as such that feminists should be opposing, but the way in which it is organized.

A critical stance, therefore, needs to be taken towards the abuse of technologies, but one that does not put the responsibility for doing this onto the childless. Of course, one of the problems here concerns the fact that the male monopoly of science and the lack of female doctors at consultant level and in positions of power (Stacey 1988, Witz 1992), mean that women have had little influence over the way in which services have been developed. For example, most research and treatment has been directed towards women, so that even when the cause of infertility lies with the male partner the female partner has been the object of treatment. As Kohler Riessman suggests: "external markers of biological processes" (1989: 212) (e.g. menstruation and lactation) make women easy targets for medical intervention, and they have no real power to challenge the status quo, or to direct research funds. However, discontinuing IVF and related technologies will not alter this state of affairs or reverse the male domination of reproduction. To call a halt to a procedure does not alter the social context in which that procedure developed in the first place. Women have not resisted the development of IVF and many have welcomed it, so that in calling for a complete halt on all treatment using IVF, radical feminists could be said to be attempting to impose their own interpretation of reality onto the majority of women.

The explanation often given for women not resisting IVF is that of false consciousness, in which women collude with men against their own ultimate interests. Certainly this study has found some instances where such an interpretation could be applied; for example, the lack of concern over drug regimes, even by women who had suffered serious side-effects, or the denial of pronatalist ideology by women who had actual experience of it. To argue, however, that women are colluding or ignorant of their true state is simply to adopt a victim-blaming approach, and one in which there can only be one interpretation of reality. As Stanley & Wise argue, feminist writing has largely ignored the fact that:

> much human behaviour cannot be described, let alone understood in unexplicated categorical terms . . . or rather resolved by treating people's experiences as faulty versions of the theoretician's categories (1990: 24).

They add that intentionally or not feminist social scientists adopting this stance place themselves as experts "on or over other women's experiences".

It is necessary, therefore, to develop mechanisms by which false consciousness can be explained without denigrating women; a situation in which women's own interpretation of their position, and of their decision making, is given value. One approach would be to construct "theory derived from experience, analytically entered into by enquiring feminists" (Stanley & Wise 1990: 24).

The radical feminist portrayal of infertile women bears many similarities to the way in which women generally are portrayed in patriarchal societies. By dismissing women's experiences as false consciousness, radical feminism is denying them just as patriarchy denies them. At the same time, by locating pronatalism as a problem of the infertile, radical feminists place considerable responsibility on the infertile to challenge it. Infertile people are a highly visible manifestation of pronatalism, but they are not its source. In its similarities to patriarchy, I would contend that radical feminism, far from liberating women, provides, for infertile women at least, an alternative form of oppression, which exploits their vulnerability in the same way as it accuses the medical profession of doing.

In contrast, it can be argued that medicine has contributed both to women's liberation and their oppression (Lupton 1994). Indeed, Kohler Riessman (1989) argues that medicalization of life problems has led to women simultaneously winning and losing. Given the range of experience and opinions of feminists it is not surprising that dilemmas and paradoxes abound in the feminist movement. As Eisenstein (1983) states, feminism is not a monolith, yet there does not seem to have been much debate that focuses at an empirical rather than a theoretical level, and which values women's own experiences of using available technology.

It is not the existence of NRTs that prevents women from having greater control over reproduction, but social, economic and political inequality. Many fears are raised by feminist writers regarding the abuse of technology, and the differential use and availability of technology, such as the idea that some women are more "suitable" mothers and therefore more "deserving" of available infertility treatment. These abuses should, of course, be of concern to us all, but the issues need to be addressed by everyone, without denigrating or putting undue pressure and responsibility on infertile women.

References

Birke, L., S. Himmelweit, G. Vines 1990. *Tomorrow's child. Reproductive technologies in the 90s*. London: Virago.

Burfoot, A. 1990. The normalisation of a new reproductive technology. In *The new reproductive technologies*, M. McNeil, I. Varcoe, S. Yearley (eds), 58–73. London: Macmillan.

Calnan, M. 1987. *Health & illness: the lay perspective*. London: Tavistock.

Calnan, M. 1988. Lay evaluation of medicine and medical practice: report of a pilot study. *International Journal of Health Services* 18, 311–22.

Cannon, S. 1989. Social research in stressful settings: difficulties of the sociologist studying the treatment of breast cancer. *Sociology of Health and Illness* 11, 62–77.

Crowe, C. 1985. Women want it: in vitro fertilization and women's motivation for participation. *Women's Studies International Forum* 8, 547–52.

Corea, G. et al. (eds) 1987. *Man made woman*. Bloomington, Indiana: Indiana University Press.

Crowe, C. 1990. Whose mind over whose matter? Women, in vitro fertilization and the development of scientific knowledge. In *The new reproductive technologies*, M. McNeil, I. Varcoe, S. Yearley (eds), 27–57. London: Macmillan.

Denny, E. 1994. Liberation or oppression? Radical feminism and in vitro fertilization. *Sociology of Health and Illness* **16**, 62–80.

Eisenstein, H. 1983. *Contemporary feminist thought*. Boston: G. K. Hall.

Franklyn, S. 1992. Making sense of missed conceptions: anthropological perspectives on unexplained infertility. In *Changing human reproduction*, M. Stacey (ed.). London: Sage.

Gabe, J. & M. Calnan 1989. The limits of medicine: women's perception of medical technology. *Social Science and Medicine* **28**, 223–31.

Graham, H. 1984. Surveying through stories. In *Social researching: politics, problems, practice*, C. Bell & H. Roberts (eds), 104–24. London: Routledge & Kegan Paul.

Hanmer, J. 1987. Reproduction trends and the production of moral panic. *Social Science and Medicine* **25**, 697–704.

Hillier, S. 1991. Women as patients & providers. In *Sociology as applied to medicine*, G. Scambler (ed.), 146–59. London: Baillière Tindall.

Holmes, H. B. & T. Tymstra 1987. In vitro fertilization in the Netherlands: experiences and opinions of Dutch women. *Journal of in vitro Fertilization and Embryo Transfer* **4**, 116–23.

Klein, R. 1987. What's new about the new reproductive technologies? In *Man made women*, G. Corea et al. (eds), 64–73. Bloomington, Indiana: Indiana University Press.

Klein, R. 1989. Resistance: from the exploitation of infertility to an explanation of infertility. In *Infertility: women speak out about their experiences of reproductive medicine*, R. Klein (ed.). London: Pandora.

Kohler Riessman, C. 1989. Women and medicalisation: a new perspective. In *Perspectives in medical sociology*, P. Brown (ed.), 190–220. Belmont, California: Wadsworth.

Lupton, D. 1994. *Medicine as culture: illness, disease and the body in western societies*. London: Sage.

Milne, B. J. 1988. Couples' experiences of in vitro fertilisation. *Journal of Obstetrics, Gynaecology and Neonatal Nursing* **17**, 347–57.

Rothman, B. K. 1984. The meaning of choice in reproductive technology. In *Test-tube women – what future for motherhood?*, R. Arditti (ed.), 22–33. London: Pandora.

Rowland, R. 1984a. Of woman born – but for how long? *Melbourne Age* 13 June 1984.

Rowland, R. 1984b. Reproductive technologies: the final solution to the woman question? In *Test-tube women – what future for motherhood?*, R. Arditti (ed.), 356–69. London: Pandora.

Rowland, R. 1985. A child at any price? *Women's Studies International Forum* **8**, 539–46.

Rowland, R. 1987a. Motherhood, patriarchal power, alienation and the issue of choice in sex pare-selection. In *Man made women*, G. Corea et al. (eds), 74–87. Bloomington, Indiana: Indiana University Press.

Rowland, R. 1987b. Technology and motherhood: reproductive choice reconsidered. *Signs* **12**, 512–29.

Sandelowski, M., B. Holditch-Davies, B. G. Harris 1990. Living the life: explanations of infertility. *Sociology of Health and Illness* **12**, 195–215.

Spallone, P. 1989. *Beyond conception: the new politics of reproduction*. London: Macmillan.

Stacey, M. 1988. *The sociology of health and healing*. London: Unwin Hyman.

Stacey, M. (ed.) 1992. *Changing human reproduction*. London: Sage.

Stanley, L & S. Wise 1990. Method, methodology and epistemology in feminist research processes. In *Feminist praxis*, L. Stanley (ed.). London: Routledge.

Stanworth, M. 1987. Reproductive technologies and the deconstruction of motherhood. In *Reproductive technologies*, M. Stanworth (ed.). Cambridge: Polity.

Steinberg, D. L. 1990. The depersonalisation of women through the administration of *in vitro* fertilisation. In *The new reproductive technologies*, M. McNeil, I. Varcoe, S. Yearley (eds), 74–142. London: Macmillan.

Strickler, J. 1992. The new reproductive technology: Problem or solution? *Sociology of Health and Illness* **14**, 111–32.

Warren, M. A. 1988. IVF and women's interests: an analysis of women's concerns. *Bioethics* **2**(1), 37–57.

Witz, A. 1992. *Professions and patriarchy*. London: Routledge.

Part V

Complementary therapies and lay re-skilling in late modernity

Chapter 11

Using complementary therapies: a challenge to orthodox medicine?

Ursula Sharma

Why do people use complementary medicine? At one level this question is scarcely worth asking since it can be answered so simply; people use complementary therapy because they feel ill and think that it will do them some good. However, given the dominance of biomedicine in this country – its virtual monopoly of the medical services provided by the state, and the fact that it is still free at the point of delivery – the straightforward and explicit question just posed carries the implicit question "why do people use complementary therapy *in preference to* orthodox medicine". In this chapter I want to address the idea that complementary medicine has come to be popular because of discontent with orthodox medicine or to fill gaps in services provided by orthodox medicine.

This view of the current popularity of complementary medicine has been voiced in various forms by the medical profession itself. For example the first BMA report, *Alternative therapies* (BMA 1986), was very negative in its assessment of the therapies themselves, but put forward the idea that their appeal is based on the ability of practitioners to spend time listening to the patient, which few doctors in the NHS as presently constituted have the time to do. Social scientists and other commentators, as we shall see later in this chapter, have put forward comparable explanations for the appeal of non-orthodox medicine, as indeed have patients themselves.

I shall address the issue at two levels. First, I will consider what we learn about patient motivation from studies of patients' choices of complementary therapy, especially in terms of changing attitudes to orthodox medicine. Here I will draw largely upon data collected in the course of research carried out by myself on users and providers of complementary therapy between 1986 and 1990. Secondly, I shall consider the question of what the increase in uptake of complementary therapy means at the public and collective level; is it evidence of some broader cultural shift in expectations about health, healing and the body, based on disillusion with the model offered by orthodox medicine? I shall argue that we must regard the rise of complementary medicine as in some measure an index of dissatisfactions with orthodox medicine, but that these dissatisfactions seem to be fairly specific, and we are not (so far) seeing a major shift away from orthodox medicine itself. Indeed, it can be argued that the rise in popularity of complementary medicine is evidence of higher expectations from medicine and healing practitioners in general, and the increasing cultural significance of the cure and care of the body in modern society.

Background: the rise of complementary medicine

Until very recently, sociologists and others who studied complementary medicine treated it as an interesting but marginal institution, supported by a "fringe" minority (Wallis & Morley 1976). Usually they situated their work in terms of the sociology of unlegitimated knowledge, deviant sects or cults. From many points of view there was nothing improper about this contextualization. But at the same time general studies of lay attitudes and illness behaviour in western societies overlooked the possibility of research subjects choosing unorthodox forms of treatment. Consequently, when it became evident in the early 1980s that increasing numbers of people were opting for unorthodox therapies of various kinds, medical sociologists and anthropologists working in western societies[1] did not have the kind of accumulated data on how and why people chose "deviant" forms of health care that would enable them to offer an immediate interpretation of this phenomenon.

The first announcements that the level of usage of non-orthodox forms of treatment was such that sociologists could not ignore them came from large-scale surveys conducted by researchers outside the academy in the late 1970s and early 1980s. It is difficult to judge the rate and areas of growth in more than a rough and ready fashion because different studies have used different methodologies and concentrated on different groups of therapies. We do not have baseline data on the rate of usage in the period before around 1975 such as would provide the starting point for longitudinal comparisons.

However, these surveys demonstrated that although use of complementary medicine was probably still a minority choice, the group who used it could not be dismissed as an insignificant "fringe". On the basis of earlier opinion polls and the results of a large-scale survey of practitioners funded by the Threshold Foundation in 1981, Stephen Fulder, a medical scientist, estimated that as many as 3.7 per cent of the adult population in Britain might be using complementary medicine in any one year (Fulder 1988). The Research Surveys of Great Britain (RSGB) poll of 1984 found that around 30 per cent of their sample had used one or more of a selection of named complementary therapies (RSGB 1984). The Market and Opinion Research International (MORI) opinion poll of 1989 found that 27 per cent of a sample of adults had used one of a selection of forms of complementary medicine at some time in their lives (MORI 1989). I do not know of any large-scale population-based studies carried out in Britain since the MORI poll. However, though we may be critical of some of the methods used and questions asked, these surveys (along with information on the increase in practitioners: Davies 1984) suggest that we should regard complementary medicine as an established feature of health care options and health care choices of people in the UK. These (by now rather old) studies suggested that a higher proportion of educated and middle-class people used complementary medicine, but that it was by no means exclusively used by the well-off. Much also depended on region, some areas of Britain (especially the London area and the southwest) being better supplied with complementary practitioners of most kinds than others. More recent research by Thomas and colleagues suggests that the proportion of women seeking treatment is still higher than that of men (63 per cent women as compared with 37 per cent men) and that complementary medicine is still relatively under-used by the very young and the very old (Thomas et al. 1991) but that the user population still appears to have a fairly broad base.

The British Medical Association's second and much more favourable report on complementary therapies (BMA 1993) was followed by a marked change in attitudes to complementary medicine in the National Health Service; changes in funding arrangements already meant that fund-holding GPs who were well disposed to a particular form or forms of complementary medicine could buy in the services of practitioners for their patients. There has been a sudden upsurge of interest in the cost effectiveness of complementary medicine among NHS managers, and it seems certain that we are about to see a further rise in usage as patients who might not have chosen complementary therapy on their own initiative as private patients obtain non-orthodox treatment via NHS gatekeepers. The material covered in this section however is largely based on data collected at a time when surveys of users of complementary medicine were interrogating mainly private patients paying for treatment obtained as a result of their own personal choice.

For what diseases or health problems is complementary medicine used? It may be hard to generalize since particular therapies may be consulted by different kinds of patients for different kinds of health problem. Osteopaths and chiropractors probably see more musculo-skeletal problems than anything else, whereas homeopaths or acupuncturists may see a wider spectrum of conditions. As use of complementary medicine becomes more widespread and as we know more about it, it becomes less and less useful to aggregate figures about therapies as different as chiropractic and spiritual healing.

Much of the existing evidence about reasons for usage comes from small-scale surveys and I have summarized much of the available information from these elsewhere (Sharma 1992: 24-5). These studies tend to show that people consult complementary medicine primarily for chronic problems of one kind and another, especially those problems for which orthodox medicine can on the whole only offer palliative care (see for instance Moore et al. 1985). There is little reason to think that people frequently rely upon complementary medicine for the treatment of acute or life-threatening conditions, though a great deal of publicity has been given to a few cases where this has happened.

The large-scale study of 2,473 patients of complementary medicine carried out by Thomas and colleagues found that 78.2 per cent were attending for musculo-skeletal problems, though this may be explained by the predominance of the patients of osteopaths and chiropractors in the sample. However, a 1993 *Daily Telegraph* survey (Doyle 1993), based on a simple poll of readers unmediated by reference to practitioners, also indicated that the biggest single category of health problems for which people consult complementary therapy is musculo-skeletal problems (60 per cent). On the face of it therefore, this kind of evidence supports the view that complementary therapy is used in areas where orthodox medicine does not "perform" well.

Patients' decisions

However, we cannot explore what the use of complementary medicine means to patients unless we move away from quantitative surveys of whatever scale, and use methods that identify both the social and clinical contexts in which patients turn to complementary medicine and allow a qualitative exploration of patients' perceptions of these situations.

Byron Good is critical of the use of choice of therapy as a method of accessing a health care system on the grounds that it is associated with an inappropriate stress on rationality:

> Although the anthropological literature on care-seeking is now quite diverse in methodology and theoretical orientation, utilitarian assumptions often appear in the commonsense reasoning in the literature. This is troubling. The analytic conjunction of the utilitarian actor, instrumental beliefs that organize the rational calculus of care-seeking, and ethnomedical systems as the sum of

strategic actions is uncomfortably consonant with neo-classical theories of the utilitarian actor, the marketplace, and the economic system as precipitate of value-maximizing strategies (Good 1994: 47).

This emphasis, he argues, discourages us from exploring the construction of meaning on the part of the patient, and leads to "an impoverished conception of human symboling". In Britain there is certainly a dearth of ethnographic studies of the cultural and moral meaning of health and illness that do not take the decision to consult a practitioner as their starting point. I admit that in my own use of this method I may have overemphasized the economic rationality of the patient. However, if we wish to explore the cultural moment at which a dominant form of healing appears to be in danger of ceding its hegemonic position, or at least when its legitimacy is seriously questioned, then we surely need to examine the circumstances in which individuals first turn to alternatives.

There are huge methodological difficulties involved in the micro study of decision making, especially where one is trying to unpick the way in which some decision has been made in retrospect. Patients' descriptions of how and why they consulted a complementary practitioner are inevitably coloured by subsequent experience of this practitioner or other complementary practitioners, the progress of the illness, and many other factors. To examine the point of choice is to isolate a moment (arbitrarily from many points of view) in what is often an ongoing story of attempts to deal with illness. The resort to the complementary practitioner becomes part of an "illness narrative" told to the researcher that may have its own current agenda (Good 1994: 135ff.; Kleinman 1988; see also Ch. 7).

Bearing in mind these methodological problems, I conducted an intensive study of 30 recent users of complementary medicine in the Stoke-on-Trent conurbation in 1986/7.[2] The interviewees were a self-selected "sample" in that they were all people who had responded to a newspaper article about my research on complementary medicine and who had offered to be interviewed. Consequently I have not used the data to speculate upon the demographic profile of complementary medicine users, nor about degrees of "satisfaction", etc. Rather I was interested to get people to tell me the "story of how they came to use complementary medicine". The interviews therefore were semi-structured, giving scope for people to tell their own stories in terms of the circumstances and events that seemed most salient to them, with prompts for certain issues that I surmised might be generally significant if the interviewees did not raise them themselves ("Did you tell your doctor you were using complementary medicine?" "Have any of your relatives used complementary medicine?"). As a result of this study I concluded, as I shall relate below, that there were several types of user in terms of the patterns of usage. In 1993 I made another small study of a group of people who might be considered "stable users" of a particular form of complementary medicine; I distributed a questionnaire to the 19 members of a homeopathic study group who met monthly at the consulting rooms of an established homeopath in a Midlands town.

From these, and from other studies that have been carried out, some general patterns emerge. First, it seems likely that few people consult a complementary practitioner about a health problem without having first presented it to an orthodox practitioner. All but one of the 30 people whom I interviewed in Stoke-on-Trent in 1986–7 had consulted their GP initially in respect of the health problem for which they first used complementary medicine. The study carried out by Kate Thomas and her colleagues found that 64 per cent of the patients studied had seen a GP or specialist before consulting a complementary practitioner about their current problem (Thomas et al. 1991). Possibly, as complementary medicine becomes better known and more acceptable, more people will use some form of complementary therapy as their first resort, but this is not the case for the majority at the moment. Orthodox medicine is first in the "hierarchy of resort" for most people, and complementary medicine is turned to when orthodox care fails or is deemed unsatisfactory from one point of view or another.

The interviewees in my own study all claimed that orthodox medicine had not been effective for the problem in hand – although we must remember that in this context "effectiveness" signifies "effective as judged by the patient". This often meant that the patient judged orthodox medical treatment capable of clearing the symptoms, but at some kind of unacceptable cost (e.g. side-effects, the treatment took too long, it involved an operation and they preferred a less drastic intervention). Here we should note the discrepancy between the kinds of judgements patients make about "efficacy" or satisfactoriness, and the kinds of criteria that orthodox medical scientists require when they insist that complementary medicine prove itself through rigorous randomized clinical trials (see, for example, the editorial in the *British Medical Journal*, 5 January 1980, entitled "The flight from science"; also BMA 1986).

Take the example of one woman who had persistent back problems:

> Dr . . . gave me an awful lot of tablets, anti-inflammatory tablets which I didn't even bother to take because I know that anti-inflammatory tablets can cause awful problems with your stomach. I have learnt this in the past.

This user of complementary medicine was not saying that the anti-inflammatory tablets would not produce relief in some measure, only that she considered that they might do so at a cost that she was not prepared to accept. Similarly, a working-class woman who had suffered from kidney trouble and high blood pressure for years had been prescribed drugs whose side-effects she found quite unacceptable:

> On those tablets I was just no-how. I could not even walk upstairs, I was that much out of breath. I was taking deep breaths in to get any air.

A herbalist, however, had treated her for some years with medicine that she found quite acceptable. She did not claim that herbal medicine was the only efficacious treatment for her condition – she accepted that no form of medicine would make her condition go away entirely and so was making a judgement on the *costs* of what was available to her.

From their own point of view, therefore, members of the orthodox profession may be right in rationalizing resort to complementary therapy in terms other than the ineffectiveness of orthodox medicine, but they are overlooking the fact that patients may not be evaluating treatments purely in terms of clinical effectiveness, but in terms of a range of quite diverse criteria.

There is certainly plenty of evidence to suggest that fear of side-effects and fear of drastic interventions is a very dominant theme in patients' decision making. For instance, in a *Daily Telegraph* poll of readers who had used complementary medicine, this was a concern of 25 per cent of the people who responded; another 52 per cent claimed that orthodox medicine was not helping them with their condition (Doyle 1993).

My own interviews with patients revealed similar anxieties. For instance, the mother of a seven-year-old stated:

> Jason had a very bad skin rash which would not clear up, and I thought it might be eczema. The doctor prescribed cortisone creams and steroids which I thought was rather drastic. We went to a homeopath who dealt with the problem more or less. It was quite a relief not to have to put cortisone cream and stuff like that all over his hands . . . I was always very worried about having medicine in the house and I was relieved that homeopathic medicines are non-poisonous. If you take a whole bottle full you are not going to die even though it may be labelled belladonna or something like that.

Similarly, a middle-aged woman who had used herbalism and acupuncture for her migraines told me:

I tried the tablets the GP gave me for my migraine. I have had all kinds, migraleve, migril, etc. which I don't believe in because they have got ergotamines and I feel the side-effects are too great and I am not prepared to risk it. I think it is much better to go that way if you can, than have all the drugs we have been taking.

Another characteristic of decisions to consult a complementary practitioner seems to be that they are mediated by the opinions of friends, relatives or neighbours. In my study of therapists carried out in 1988–90 in a Midlands locality, almost all the practitioners claimed that a major source of patients was the local grapevine. This is in line with the results of earlier research, such as Peter Davies's study of practitioners, which suggests that 73 per cent of referrals come by word of mouth (Davies 1984: 20). My own data suggest that the decision to consult a particular complementary practitioner seems to be a product of (mainly) local lay referral networks. Consider, for instance, the following extracts from interviews:

I found out (about the practitioner that I used) from a colleague of my husband's. His wife had liver cancer. She was given four weeks to live four years ago and she is still alive now. He told my husband about it, he said just get on the phone and ring her (woman suffering from difficult menopausal symptoms).

I have a friend who was studying acupuncture. She saw that I was struggling more than I should be and she suggested to me that we see X (an established acupuncturist). In fact she took me to see him herself (young man suffering from chronic fatigue and depression).

My mother-in-law who lived in London had a friend whose daughter had very similar back problems to mine. She suggested this osteopath to me and that was how I started to use osteopathy (women with chronic back pain).

This reliance on personal networks seems to be in part due to the lack of other sources of information, and in part a reflection of a need for the first trial of an unfamiliar treatment to be with someone who could be vouched for by a member of the sick person's local community. In the late 1980s, referrals from GPs seem to have been unusual, in spite of studies of GPs and medical students showing positive attitudes to complementary medicine (Wharton & Lewith 1986, Furnham 1993). The General Medical Council had in 1977 removed the prohibition on GPs making such referrals provided that they still maintained overall therapeutic responsibility for the patient, so official professional barriers to such referrals have been long gone. Possibly the problem for GPs was how to exert responsibility in practice when referring patients to practitioners outside the NHS with whom they had no official channels of communication (see Sharma 1992 for a discussion of this problem).

Patterns of usage

In as much as patients appear to be taking the initiative in seeking different kinds of health care, and judging it in terms of value for money, their behaviour can be described as "consumerist". Not surprisingly, the medical profession has regarded patient "consumerism" with, at best, great caution (see the BMJ editorial "The flight from science", 5 January 1980). Possibly the attitude of those who had money to spend on health care has always been "consumerist" in this sense. The main difference between the situation described by Roy Porter in regard to "quacks" and commercial cures and therapies in the seventeenth and eighteenth centuries (Porter 1994) and the situation today is that the modern health care consumer has more sources of information about the different systems of therapy, especially those derived from the media.

Certainly some of the people I interviewed explicitly espoused a "consumerist" view of their choices. One interviewee described how, as a result of her experience in using homeopathy for rhinitis, she had developed a greater confidence in her own capacity to judge the kind of therapy which would be best for particular problems she experienced:

> I make up my own mind about these things now. Now I feel I am
> in control of my life.

She went on to castigate those who, though they have the money for health care available, begrudge paying £20 for helpful therapy but will spend the same amount on a meal or an evening at the theatre.

The problem of looking at individual decisions to use complementary medicine in terms of consumer choice, however, is that such decisions do not take place in isolation but as part of chains of decision making. For a start, they take place within the context of the history of a particular illness or health problem. Looking at the issue from a wider perspective, a person who uses complementary medicine may do so as a "one-off" decision in respect of a particular illness. Alternatively, they may do so as part of an established general preference (on the part of either individual or household) for a particular therapy. Or (as in the case of the woman just quoted) they may show an emerging tendency towards eclecticism in choice of health care. Therefore in my study I tried to situate the decision to consult, which I had asked patients to talk about in detail, within a current pattern of practice (without any assumption of course that such a pattern would continue without changing). Looking at the data in this way, a number of patterns emerged from this rather small sample (see Figure 11.1).

From the diagram it can be seen that only eight of the sample used complementary medicine alone for most health problems. These included

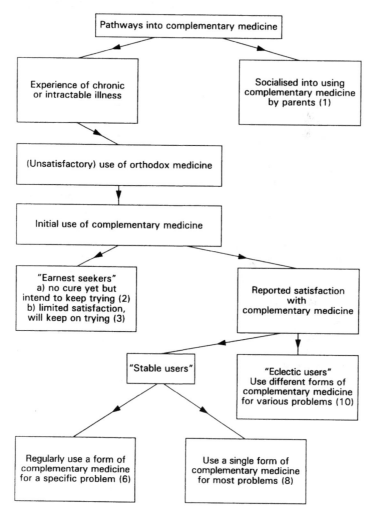

Figure 11.1 How people use complementary medicine: patterns of practice. Adapted from Sharma, *Complementary medicine today* (London: Routledge, 1992).

a couple of people who could really be regarded as the products of an earlier wave of alternative practice, people who had turned to homeopathy or naturopathy in the inter-war period. The others were usually people who had found a particular practitioner in whose therapy and personal skill they had great faith. I have termed "eclectic users" the group who used complementary therapy frequently, but with no settled loyalty to a particular therapy or therapist. The rest of the interviewees were people whose use of complementary medicine was presently dominated by the need to resolve a particular pressing health problem. I have termed "earnest seekers" those who had not found any therapy that entirely solved their problem at the time of the interview but who intended to keep on trying. The six interviewees who regularly used a particular therapy for a particular problem had found a form of treatment that they felt was tackling a specific problem with good results (probably former "earnest seekers"). What a study like this cannot tell us of course is how many or what sort of people cease their "earnest seeking", unsatisfied with any of the options they have tried.

None of the interviewees said that they could think of *no* situations in which they might use orthodox medicine. Those that spoke of eclectic consumerism, value for money (mainly the "earnest seekers" and the "eclectic users") were not excluding orthodox medicine from the range of therapies from which they made choices. In my 1993 study of "stable users", all expressing deep commitment to homeopathy, 17 of the 19 respondents could cite visits to their GPs within the past year and the remaining two could think of occasions when they had visited their GP during the past three years. Indeed the literature on patients' usage of complementary medicine generally confirms that not only is it unusual for people who use complementary medicine to have abandoned orthodox medicine altogether, but it is not uncommon for patients to use both systems simultaneously for the same problem (24 per cent of those in Thomas et al.'s study, for example). A Dutch study published in 1981 (Ooijendijk et al. 1981) showed that very few people in a sample of users of complementary medicine had not visited their GP in the previous year (15 per cent) whereas as many as 32 per cent had visited three to seven times and 22 per cent had visited eight times or more. That is, there was a substantial category of people who were high users of *both* kinds of medicine (see also Murray & Shepherd 1993).

This parallel usage was reflected in my interviews. For example, a factory inspector spoke of the use that he and his wife had made of reflexology and herbalism, and the changes they had made in their family diet:

We get a lot of ideas from our friends (who use whole foods) and there is a lot more information on TV and so forth. If we need to, we do go to our GP. We are not totally blinkered. We are not totally dedicated to alternative medicine. We aim to get the best from both systems.

Another interviewee, a woman suffering from severe migraines, had used homeopathic remedies that, she said, had been effective in reducing the frequency and severity of attacks to some extent. However, she continued to receive prescriptions from her GP for drugs that she used occasionally when the pain was very severe.

Perceptions of complementary therapists and doctors

This did not mean that users of complementary medicine saw their dependence on more than one system of healing as unproblematic. Most (60 per cent) avoided the possibility of censure from their GPs by simply not telling them that they were using other forms of healing. Few wished to make drastic criticisms of their own GPs' services, but perhaps it is inevitable that plural usage leads to greater reflection upon the nature of the service offered by the GP, even if this is not the issue that has precipitated use of complementary medicine. Though only one interviewee reported a real breakdown in her relationship with her GP, several commented on the unsatisfactory nature of GP/patient relations in general and compared them unfavourably with the relationship they felt they enjoyed with a complementary therapist. For example, a teacher who had used a variety of therapies for himself and his children said:

If a homeopath or a herbalist treats the patient they tend to explain. I have seen little old ladies in the chemist shop ask the chemist things because they are afraid to ask the doctor, to take up more of his time.

A community worker who had a very conflictual relationship with her GP commented on her family's experience of orthodox and complementary health care:

I think [the GP] just had it in for us. We were trouble. But we liked the homeopathic doctor and I don't think it was just because she was being paid. What she seemed to do was to relate to us all as people. That was the nice thing. She was interested in knowing how we lived, so that she could assess the broad influences on our health. GPs object to you going in and saying things like "we think we have got so-and-so, we don't want chemical drugs necessarily but could you tell us what it is?" They want you to be more passive.

The comment that the complementary therapist had more time to talk about health problems than GPs was a recurrent theme in both the interviews and the questionnaire responses (see also Murray & Shepherd 1993). Frankenberg has noted that in the intersection between the patient's own biographical time and the biomedical doctor's clinical time there is a struggle for control in which biomedicine, through the constraints and the disciplines of the clinic, has the advantage (Frankenberg 1992). Many of the complementary practitioners whom I interviewed in a later study expressed doubts as to whether they could provide the same sort of unpressured service to patients if they were incorporated into the NHS and subjected to its more bureaucratic conceptions of the cost-effective use of time (Sharma 1992: 142ff.; see also Cant & Calnan 1991). Yet this is clearly what many patients value about the service offered by complementary therapists. For example Lilian,[3] a retired teacher, contrasted the way in which her GP and her acupuncturist had dealt with her cancer. While appreciating the speed with which her GP obtained a referral for her, and the efficiency with which the specialist organized her treatment, she noted their impersonality in dealing with her:

> Everyone said he [GP] is a good man, you are lucky and I got in quite quickly [for a mastectomy], but neither he nor the specialist offered me a single word of advice or comfort or encouragement – not a word. They didn't tell me about the success rate of the operation – you don't want false hopes but you do need encouragement.

After the operation the acupuncturist treated her for "tension":

> He [acupuncturist] gave me good advice and he said get lots of rest and fresh air – obvious things really, but it is nice to have them said.

Similarly, John, a young man with a chronic condition of the scalp, who had tried homeopathy (too recently to pronounce about the degree of success of the treatment) commented:

> They [complementary practitioners] give you more time. Obviously most of them charge you, so they would do. But most of them treat the individual symptoms as the individual's *problem*, not just as a Latinized term. Whereas my doctor, he just seems to dip into his little book of medications.

Some interviewees noted that complementary therapists not only had more time but were more informative, more inclined to take an educational approach to health care. Dave, a music teacher suffering from chronic ear infections as well as migraines and complex psychological problems, expressed appreciation of the herbalist who had been treating him for some months:

> When I saw her I thought, she is of my intelligence, she treats me as an equal. She convinced me that it is the whole of my body [that is problematic]. The dietary advice she gave me was [in order] to change my metabolism . . . You have to study your own metabolism and this I had never done. I had to do a massive questionnaire about my family background. No-one had ever asked me to do this before. I had to ring up my mother and go back to bronchial asthma in my family before the turn of the century . . . all this seemed to come back together and it was *my* body and *my* temperament.

Dave expressed some anger at the way his GP had treated his case since he felt that the doctor had been too ready to prescribe antibiotics without looking at what he had learnt to regard as the deep-seated causes of these recurrent infections.

To summarize this section of the chapter, the detailed examination of the choices of a small sample of users of complementary medicine suggests that the figures generated by large-scale surveys may mask a variety of patterns of usage, which we have no reason to assume to be stable. Although a few users of complementary medicine may abandon orthodox medicine, or at any rate regard it as strictly for use in the case of a life-threatening emergency, it is clear that a larger number continue to use orthodox medicine in one way or another, while retaining a critical stance towards certain aspects of orthodox practice. The problem of interpreting the rise of complementary medicine in general terms is therefore bound to be a complex task.

Interpreting cultural change: the wider scene

The search for meaning

This is the point at which the choices of complementary therapy that occur in personal narratives and household histories about illness and how it is dealt with need to be inserted into stories about what is happening to modern industrial societies, about the forms of health care they favour and pay for, and the relationship between different systems of health care in the same polity.

Some medical anthropologists, in line with the current emphasis on anthropology as the study of meaning, have tended to look at different forms of healing in terms of the ways in which they provide meaning to sufferers rather than in terms of what clinical results they might be held to affect. In as much as the use of complementary medicine (at present) occurs mainly in the context of chronic illness and, in as much as chronic illness often presents particular threats to the integrity of a person's social identity, to ask how complementary medicine might compare with conventional medicine in its interpretive capacity seems a very pertinent question.

Cecil Helman for instance has suggested (and presumably he is drawing on his experience as a GP as well as his anthropological insight) that patients appreciate complementary medicine because it is good at giving meaning to suffering:

> Many patients have an unfulfilled sense of wanting to be connected, once again, to some wider context, to locate their suffering in a wider framework – even to somehow contain within themselves the many cycles of nature . . . Complementary practitioners often help people "make sense" of their situation in a more meaningful way than does medicine, often utilizing more traditional modes of dealing with human misfortune . . . many of them utilize traditional cultural beliefs in order to explain to the patient why they have been affected by that particular illness at that particular time (Helman 1992: 12).

This is in keeping with the tendency of medical anthropology to see perceptions of illness in a wider context than systems of belief about health and illness, a context that gives moral meaning to misfortune and suffering of diverse kinds and links personal concerns with the individual body to wider collective concerns. Carol MacCormack, for instance, sees the movement for holistic healing as possibly a response to alienation, perhaps "a viable response to the psychic numbing engendered by the enormities of our time" (MacCormack 1991: 269).

From the data provided by my own study, I would say that there is likely to be considerable truth in what Helman surmises, but that we must be careful not to romanticize the quest for meaning. Some of the people I interviewed certainly commented on complementary practitioners' ability to help them make sense of their illness in a broader way than did conventional medicine, but they seemed to be referring to explanations of symptoms – answers to the question "*what* is happening to me?" rather than answers to the question "*why* should this suffering happen to me of all people?"

This is not a theme that respondents in either of my studies raised of their own accord. Several did, however, refer to the therapist providing them with a new way of looking at their health problems; a new context in which to understand their symptoms. Thus Dave, quoted in the previous section, is inspired by the fact that his herbalist can reveal a consistency of experience, a profile of diverse health problems that turn out to be related to his family background, to his environment and lifestyle, and to his personal constitution. The apparently random symptoms that the GP had been treating in an ad hoc manner were now revealed to be part of a pattern. We can call this "making sense", but is this to say any more than that the practitioner has given the patient a full and clear explanation of symptoms in terms of the knowledge framework within which she practices her discipline? A sensitive GP might do the same though, as we have already seen, time is the very thing that GPs are perceived as either lacking or not wishing to devote to patients' queries and understanding of their health problems.

Changing health beliefs

Adrian Furnham, a psychologist, has wrestled with the problem of how far patients' resort to complementary medicine is actually motivated by cultural models of health and illness that are *already* different from the models that conventional medicine offers. One of his studies compared two groups of patients, a sample of those attending a GP's surgery and one of patients consulting a medically qualified homeopath. Differences in cultural conviction between these groups of patients proved to be slight, the more important differences being experience of illness and treatment; those who consulted a complementary practitioner did so out of practical frustration with unsatisfactory orthodox treatment for their (mainly chronic) health problems (Furnham & Smith 1988).

In a comparable study of users of both orthodox and complementary medicine for pain, Kelvinson and Payne found significant differences between the two groups, with the users of complementary medicine believ(ing) themselves to be responsible for their own health, being less fatalistic and trusting more in themselves than in orthodox medicine, than those patients receiving more conventional treatments (Kelvinson & Payne 1993: 5).

The results of such studies are confusing, and Kelvinson and Payne are probably right in referring to Finnigan's conclusion that users of complementary medicine are a heterogeneous group (Finnigan 1991), some of whom may consult because they hold particular health ideologies whereas others consult for purely pragmatic reasons related to particular symptoms. But, as Furnham and Smith suggest, even those who do not initially consult a complementary practitioner out of any special conviction may, as a result of exposure to the ideas of a particular therapist, come to change notions that they previously held. My study of complementary practitioners suggests that many do see the education of the patient as part of their therapeutic work and that they do spend time explaining some aspects of what they are trying to achieve with the patient (Sharma 1992: 170ff.). Patient interviews confirmed this, as the case of Dave (discussed earlier) indicates, though that is not to say that patients necessarily understood the therapy in precisely the same way as the therapist.

I have spent some time discussing this topic because I think that we should be cautious about assuming that new cultural ideas about the body, health and healing as expressed by practitioners (or identified by social scientists) are automatically shared by patients. When social scientists test the conviction of the users themselves a rather different picture emerges, which suggests we should be cautious about hailing major cultural shifts.

The medical encounter

Possibly the main changes have been in concepts of the patient's role in creating health and treating illness, and in the kind of expectations patients entertain about practitioners of any persuasion (Sharma 1994). Rosemary Taylor, for instance, sees the popularity of complementary medicine as a response to disillusionment with the "medical encounter". Taylor's argument is that orthodox medicine resisted the political demand for greater participation and democratization that emerged in the 1960s and 1970s (and which affected other professions and institutions besides medicine). Unsatisfied demand for more patient participation and more specific dissatisfactions with the still very hierarchical medical conception of the patient–practitioner relationship led some patients to choose the "exit" option – to turn to non-orthodox forms of healing. Indeed this relationship has probably deteriorated overall, with less trust and confidence in doctors, not to mention the "malpractice crisis". Taylor sees complementary medicine therefore in the context of shifts in *political* rather than *medical* culture (Taylor 1984).

Looking at the issue in these terms, the interviewees cited above are not really expressing any very novel criticisms of the NHS. What is notable is their preparedness to act on their dissatisfactions and to have the confidence to seek out some unfamiliar form of practice in the hope that it will prove better.

Some commentators might query the assumption implied in Taylor's work (and that of many others), namely that there was a period when "orthodox medicine ruled OK" as arch-modernist institution, with general acknowledgement of its claims to central authority over discourses about health and illness, as well as real power over the determination of healing activities. Thus Bakx (1991) cautiously places his analysis of the demand for complementary medicine within a discussion of the emergence of a postmodernist questioning of the modernist project, but he rejects the idea that there ever was a mass cultural consensus. Therefore he uses the term "eclipse" rather than "demise" to refer to the period when non-orthodox forms of medicine were less significant as a sector of health care in countries like Britain (Bakx 1991).

The rise in complementary medicine: continuity or radical break?

Thus far the rise of complementary medicine has been discussed largely in terms of perceptions of the shortcomings of orthodox medicine and certainly there is much in the body of research on individual use of complementary medicine that supports this view, provided that we bear in mind that the said shortcomings of orthodox medicine are probably very heterogeneous.

But one could argue there is a sense in which this is too obvious a conclusion to be interesting, one that only gets taken seriously because orthodox medicine has for so long convinced us all (social scientists included) that it can provide total health care, and that any other system must be either quackery or based on culturally eccentric notions about health, sickness and the body. In actual practice any system of medicine will generate some failures and dissatisfactions, nothing will both please and cure all the patients all the time. There is a sense in which many current patients of particular complementary therapies could just as well be said to be dissatisfied patients of other complementary therapies, in as much as some have not only tried orthodox medicine and been dissatisfied but have also already tried other forms of complementary medicine unsuccessfully. The more different forms of health care are available, the more there will be circulation of patients among them, some patients probably never finding the cure they are looking for.

This raises the question of how useful it is to look purely at the "demand" side of the equation. Instead of asking why people choose complementary medicine when it is available (why shouldn't they, if no one system can cure everyone?), we should be asking how it is that so many more different forms of medicine are available now than was the case 20 years ago, i.e. look at the "supply" side of the equation.

There are some very prosaic answers to this question, such as the possibility that we are really seeing an economic rather than a medical phenomenon. People who are in employment have more disposable income than they did in the immediate post-war period and some of them will decide to use some of this money on experimenting with different kinds of health care, both orthodox and complementary. The rise of complementary medicine can therefore be seen as an aspect of the increased provision of private medicine.

Another approach however, which is quite compatible with these mundane considerations but which does not throw the issue of the meaning of suffering, illness and healing out of the window altogether, is Rosalind Coward's suggestion that the rise of complementary medicine is an aspect of a very broad cultural shift that has to do with attitudes to the body in general, not just ideas about appropriate forms of healing (Coward 1989). Complementary medicine, she argues, is based on the idea of perfect health of mind and body as an achievable aim. Indeed it is regarded not just as an aim that is achievable but one that we should feel *obliged* to strive for. If we do not make efforts to attain it, if we cling to our "need to be ill", then we are denying the opportunity for complete fulfilment at the mental, spiritual and physical levels. This holistic perspective places responsibility for health entirely on the individual. Often it is associated with a model of the patient–practitioner relationship in which patients are led towards a mature responsibility for their own healing, and the healer guides them in that process rather than simply delivering a cure that the patient may or may not understand or participate in.

> The body has a whole new centrality as a place of work and transformation . . . Only with deep health will we be truly immune, exempt from attacks of illness and untouchable by the stresses and strains of modern life. And our minds and emotions are described as being ultimately in control of these transformations; it is up to us to make the choice to be well and that choice will be reflected in the state of our immunity (Coward 1989: 194).

On the whole this model represents, she says, a conservative or at any rate anti-collectivist ideological tendency, one that is liable to encourage victim blaming in the case of therapeutic failure. It is not one that favours real empowerment of patients as she understands empowerment, which would depend on an effective social and political analysis of the causes of ill health.

Coward focuses on the ideology of complementary medicine as she depicts it (and her depiction is based on the claims of practitioners rather than on reported patient views of what it means to them). Coward could therefore be criticized on the grounds that she has not demonstrated that patients actually chose complementary medicine because they agree with the claims she outlines, or indeed are affected by them in any way.

It is notoriously difficult to make effective theoretical links between ideas or concepts current in public representations and discourse and the choices and decision of individuals (as we can see from the debate about the effects on children of video nasties that has got bogged down in the problem of isolating a causal relationship between representation and behaviour). However, perhaps it is not essential to Coward's argument to show that patients actually agree with the ideological claims of therapists, only that these claims, when they encounter them, appeal to them enough for them to try the therapies (or to go on using them).

Conclusion

To summarize the argument so far, I have discussed much evidence that suggests that the use of complementary medicine is – indeed to some extent must be – related to dissatisfactions with orthodox medicine. The rise of complementary medicine is bound to tell us something about the way in which orthodox medicine is understood and perceived. Yet the dissatisfactions and doubts expressed by users of complementary therapies (for instance, fears about side-effects of drugs, dissatisfactions with delays in the NHS) are ones that we know about already because they have been widely identified and discussed (see Calnan 1987). How *radical* then, is the dissatisfaction that the rise of complementary medicine represents?

One way of looking at the popularity of complementary medicine is to see it in terms of the rise of a countersystem, dialectically opposed to orthodox medicine with its medical scientific paradigm and stress on hierarchical relations between the practitioner/scientist and layperson/ patient. In Lyng's analysis, the holistic health movement and several other broad cultural models of health (e.g. the public health model and what he calls the biopsychosocial model of health), all emphasize the interdependence of individual organism and environment and suggest a model of healing and health that stresses an active stance towards health, patients seeking out the kinds of knowledge or therapy that will help them achieve good health and avoid dysfunction. This countersystem, it should be noted, is a "constructed type" built up from various empirical elements; part of a dialectical understanding of modern health care systems. It need not exist in this precise form to act as reference point in analyzing shifts in what both practitioners and patients are doing and saying (Lyng 1988).

Complementary healers themselves have certainly drawn upon such a paradigm, or at any rate those who have seen their best professional bet as stressing their distinctiveness from orthodox medicine have done so. Others, like the osteopaths and chiropractors, have sought medical approval in carving out a market niche for the treatment of specific types of problem for which orthodox medicine does not have much of a reputation. As we have seen, some patients will certainly draw on such a dialectical paradigm when they discuss their decisions to consult, or their reactions to the consultation retrospectively, though we cannot assume that this is universal.

Looking at the move towards pluralism in health care as evidence of postmodernism or as part of a dialectical opposition is to emphasize diversity and difference at the expense of continuity. But suppose instead we decide to emphasize historical continuity and cultural consistency over time? Rather than representing either the stuff of a countersystem or the breakdown of yet another modernist metanarrative, suppose we regard complementary medicine as yet another transformation of a particular set of distinctively western concerns with the individual and the body. Both Coward (1989) and Crawford (1980), have emphasized the concern of holistic medicine with the individual – not just as an object of therapy (most therapy in western societies has the individual person as its object) but with individuals as the source of their own diseases. Not only is

> Self or individual responsibility . . . the mechanism believed to propel the transition from a medically dominated experience to one more meaningful, autonomous and effective for health maintenance and promotion

but

> the failure to maintain health is ascribed to some kind of willingness to be well or an unconscious desire to be sick, or simply a failure of will . . . the no-fault principle contained in the classical sick role formulation, itself a forgery, is being withdrawn. It is being replaced by a "your fault" dogma (Crawford 1980: 379).

Healthism de-medicalizes personal health in as much as it encourages the individual to be less dependent on orthodox medical direction yet paradoxically it engages in a re-medicalization of life, redefining happiness and wellbeing in general as an issue of health that the individual must address or be guilty of irresponsibility. Thus "healthism" as depicted by Crawford is a pervasive phenomenon, fuelling the self-care movement as well as recourse to holistic healing – two institutional manifestations of a general ideological tendency.

Although these movements present a challenge to orthodox medicine, the ideological premises on which they are built are not foreign to orthodox medicine, for orthodox medicine itself is based on a form of individualism in which

> in escaping from a nosology of morbid essences, [it] builds its science and clinical practice on the closed grounds of what becomes in principle an observed occurrence within the individual body (Crawford 1980: 371).

But not the body politic, for this ideology effectively denies a collective and social dimension of health; a genuinely social epidemiology.

So from this point of view, not only is complementary therapeutic thought and practice continuous with other broad reactions to the role of biomedicine in modern society such as the self-care movement, it actually perpetuates some aspects of the ideology of biomedicine itself. As Crawford notes, ideology is defined as much by the moral options that are overlooked and omitted as by what is addressed and elaborated, and while holism may do much to empower the individual, neither it nor orthodox medical ideology offer ways of empowering social action to improve the conditions in which people live and suffer ill health.

In these terms complementary medicine can be seen as an aspect of a wider cultural scene of which orthodox medicine is also a part, its popularity driven by factors that affect orthodox medicine as well, and which do not invariably drive patients away from orthodox medicine. Complementary medicine draws on (or is fuelled by, if we prefer to look at it in this way) the modern moralistic concern with the perfectibility of the body, and the individual's responsibility for its imperfections. But so do many other discourses about the body, many of which are quite consistent with the concerns and knowledge base of modern medical science – fitness regimes, cosmetic surgery, preventive medicine, and so on. All these practices exemplify what Shilling has called "body projects":

> . . . accepting that its appearance, size, shape and even its contents are potentially open to reconstruction in line with the designs of its owner . . . it (involves) individuals' being conscious of and actively concerned about the management, maintenance and appearance of their bodies (Shilling 1993: 5).

Looking at complementary medicine from this point of view it represents a set of practices that, although novel to some extent, manifest cultural concerns that have a wider relevance and which equally have their counterparts in biomedicine.

Going further, we could remind ourselves yet again that use of complementary medicine is not associated with widespread abandonment of orthodox medicine. Indeed in spite of criticisms of orthodox medicine such as those cited here, there has been widespread alarm at the idea that orthodox medicine as supported by the state in the form of the NHS might be under threat. Enthusiastic use of complementary medicine appears to go alongside ever increasing use of orthodox medicine. Possibly this is but one aspect of a cultural concern with health, a general tendency to see the healers (in general) as holding key answers to moral concerns. We may be turning more and more to holistic healers who have low status in relation to highly paid and socially powerful doctors, but we are still expecting to turn to healers of various kinds for the solution to personal problems of a wide diversity – as opposed to say, religious leaders, or to not seeking professional help at all but relying on family and social network resources. And, returning to the concerns of Helman and Kleinman cited earlier, why should people expect healers to provide them with meaning for their suffering (as opposed to other kinds of ideologue)? If people seek such meanings from healers, does this not imply that they are unable to construct such ideas themselves, or have no agreed current folk theodicies available? Seen from this point of view both the rise of complementary medicine and the continued concern with orthodox medicine appear as twin aspects of a dominant concern with health and the body, and a dominant expectation that it will be professional experts who deliver health and happiness, or at least the prerequisites for its achievement.

Looking at the issue from this point of view we could say that the use of complementary medicine offers the patient a means of expressing criticism of orthodox medicine, but one that exists within the same cultural paradigm. With increasing acceptance of certain forms of complementary medicine it is highly likely that orthodox medicine will accommodate some practices that are now regarded as complementary medicine within its own fold (as seems to be happening with osteopathy and chiropractic and has already happened with certain forms of homeopathy).

When we examine use of complementary medicine at the level of individual choice we are aware of the contrasting nature of complementary and orthodox medicine, because we are asking patients to say why they chose the one and not the other. Naturally they will specify what they think the differences are, and this is indeed instructive. It does not, however, tell us why the use of orthodox medicine remains high. Nor does it tell us why, while there are now calls for complementary medicine to be provided on the NHS, there is no call for a reduction in orthodox medical services. Indeed during and since the last election there has been much public anxiety about possible threats to the NHS.

There is an enormous interest in things medical and very high expectations of modern medicine. There is also a high level of media interest in medical issues and lay people can become quite knowledgeable about advances in medicine on the basis of information provided in popular publications, TV programmes, and so on – what Giddens (1991) has referred to as "lay re-skilling" (see Chs 1, 4 and 12). I do not think we need take this interest in orthodox medicine as self-explanatory. Rosalind Coward could be right about the popularity of complementary medicine being related to a particular form of modern moral focus on the individual's responsibility for a perfectible body. The difference in emphasis between complementary medicine and orthodox medicine is that the former stresses private and voluntary acceptance of responsibility (positive striving for health, seen as a process of moral development) whereas much orthodox discourse stresses self-responsibility as the duty of the cost-conscious citizen, and may even seek to enforce such a notion (e.g. recent controversial decisions to withhold treatment from people who smoke or are overweight). But even so, the concerns that produce popularity of complementary medicine on the part of patients seem closely related to the concerns that produce interest in and about the provision of orthodox medicine.

The choice between these two ways of looking at complementary medicine (dialectical countersystem versus manifestation of general preoccupation with the individual body? Herald of a new form of health care versus evidence of cultural continuity?) is not a matter of finding a fit with empirical facts, but a matter of choice of perspective or focus. I use these visual terms advisedly. When we focus on something near to, as we might when looking through a microscope or just an ordinary magnifying glass, we see it very differently from the way we would if a photograph were taken through a wide angle or telescopic lens. The focus on the individual's decision to use complementary medicine tells us much about changing perceptions/expectations of different kinds of healing. Focusing on the broader cultural canvas enables us to ask questions about the role of healing in general in our society and compare it with other societies or other periods of time. Which perspective we choose depends on what theoretical problems we want to resolve by asking the question "why do people use complementary medicine"?

Notes

1. In this chapter I have dealt almost exclusively with data from studies carried out in Britain. However, studies conducted in the United States (e.g. Eisenberg et al. 1993), Australia (Boven et al. 1977) and various European

countries (Sermeus 1987) suggest that very little that I have said here would not be applicable in other western countries.

2. This study was funded by a Small Grant from the Nuffield Foundation, which I acknowledge with gratitude. Thanks are also due to Sarah Cant for many interesting discussions of complementary medicine that have helped me to clarify my thinking on this subject.

3. I have used pseudonyms when referring to interviewees by name.

References

Bakx, K. 1991. The "eclipse" of folk medicine in western society? *Sociology of Health and Illness* **13**(1), 20–38.

Boven, R., C. Genn, G. Lupton, S. Payne, M. Sheehan, J. Western 1977. *New patients to alternative medicine. Western report no 1*. Appendix to Report of the Committee of Enquiry on Chiropractic, Osteopathy, Homoeopathy and Naturopathy. Parliamentary Paper No 102, Government of Australia.

British Medical Association (BMA) 1986. *Alternative therapy*. Report of the Board of Science and Education. London: BMA.

British Medical Association (BMA) 1993. *Complementary medicine. New approaches to good practice*. Oxford: Oxford University Press.

Calnan, M. 1987. *Health and illness. The lay perspective*. London: Tavistock.

Cant, S. & M. Calnan 1991. On the margins of the market place? An exploratory study of alternative practitioners' perceptions. *Sociology of Health and Illness* **13**(1), 39–57.

Coward, R. 1989. *The whole truth. The myth of alternative health*. London: Faber & Faber.

Crawford, R. 1980. Healthism and the medicalization of everyday life. *International Journal of Health Services* **10**(3), 365–88.

Davies, P. 1984. *Report on trends in complementary medicine*. London: Institute of Complementary Medicine.

Doyle, C. 1993. Reaching out for an alternative. *Daily Telegraph* 6 April 1993 p. 19.

Eisenberg, D., R. C. Kessler, C. Foster, F. E. Norlock, D. R. Calkins, D. Delbanco 1993. Unconventional medicine in the United States. *New England Journal of Medicine* **328**(4), 246–51.

Finnigan, M. D. 1991. The Centre for the Study of Complementary Medicine: an attempt to understand its popularity through psychological, demographic and operational criteria. *Complementary Medical Research* **5**(2), 83–7.

Frankenberg, R. 1992. Your time or mine? In *Time, health and medicine*, R. Frankenberg (ed.), 1–30. London: Sage.

Fulder, S. 1988. *The handbook of complementary medicine*, 2nd edn. Sevenoaks: Coronet Books.

Furnham, A. 1993. Attitudes to alternative medicine: a study of the perceptions of those studying orthodox medicine. *Complementary Therapies in Medicine* **1**(3), 120–26.

Furnham, A & C. Smith 1988. Choosing alternative medicine: a comparison of the beliefs of patients visiting a GP and a homoeopath. *Social Science and Medicine* 26(7), 685–9.

Giddens, A. 1991. *Modernity and self identity.* Cambridge: Polity.

Good, B. 1994. *Medicine, rationality and experience. An anthropological perspective.* Cambridge: Cambridge University Press.

Helman, C. 1992. Complementary medicine in context. *Medical World* 9, 11–12.

Kelvinson, R. & S. Payne 1993. Decision to seek complementary medicine for pain: a controlled study. *Complementary Therapies in Medicine* 1(1), 2–5.

Kleinman, A. 1988. *The illness narratives.* New York: Basic Books.

Lyng, S. 1988. *Holistic health and biomedicine. A countersystem analysis.* New York: State University of New York Press.

Market and Opinion Research International (MORI) 1989. *Research on alternative medicine* (conducted for *The Times* newspaper).

MacCormack, C. 1991. Holistic health and a changing western world view. In *Anthropologies of medicine. A colloquium on West European and North American perspectives*, B. Pfleiderer & G. Bibeau (eds), 259–73. Braunschweig: Vieweg.

Moore, J., K. Phipps, D. Marcer 1985. Why do people seek treatment by alternative medicine? *British Medical Journal* 290, 28–9.

Murray, J. & S. Shepherd 1993. Alternative or additional medicine? An exploratory study in general practice. *Social Science and Medicine* 37(8), 983–8.

Ooijendijk, W., J. Mackenbach, H. Limberger 1981. *What is better?* Netherlands Institute of Preventive Medicine, and The Technical Industrial Organisation. London: translated and published by the Threshold Foundation.

Porter, R. 1994. Quacks: an unconscionable time dying. In *The healing bond. Therapeutic responsibility and the patient–practitioner relationship*, S. Budd & U. Sharma (eds), 63–81. London: Tavistock/Routledge.

Research Surveys of Great Britain (RSGB) 1984. *Omnibus survey on alternative medicine* (prepared for Swan House Special Events).

Sermeus, G. 1987. *Alternative medicine in Europe. A quantitative comparison of the use and knowledge of alternative medicine and patient profiles in nine European countries.* Brussels: Belgian Consumers' Association.

Sharma, U. 1992. *Complementary medicine today. Practitioners and patients.* London: Tavistock/Routledge.

Sharma, U. 1994. The equation of responsibility: complementary practitioners and their patients. In *The healing bond. Therapeutic responsibility and the patient–practitioner relationship*, S. Budd & U. Sharma (eds), 82–103. London: Tavistock/Routledge.

Shilling, C. 1993. *The body and social theory.* London: Sage.

Taylor, C. R. 1984. Alternative medicine and the medical encounter in Britain and the United States. In *Alternative medicine. Popular and policy perspectives*, J. Warren Salmon (ed), 191–228. London: Tavistock.

Thomas, K., J. Carr, L. Westlake, B. Williams 1991. Use of non-orthodox and conventional health care in Great Britain. British Medical Journal 302, 207–10.

Wallis, R. & P. Morley (eds) 1976. *Marginal medicine.* London: Peter Owen.

Wharton, R. & G. Lewith 1986. Complementary medicine and the general practitioner. *British Medical Journal* 292, 1498–5000.

Chapter 12

Conclusions: modern medicine and the lay populace in late modernity

Simon J. Williams & Michael Calnan

At the beginning of this book we posed three main questions that the volume as a whole sought to address. First, how do lay people view modern medicine and what is the nature of their experiences of medical care and technology? Secondly, what criteria do lay people draw upon and what are the factors that shape and influence their evaluations of modern medicine? Finally, at a broader level, what does all this tell us about the relationship between modern medicine and the lay populace in the contemporary era and what light does it shed on the more macro-focused theoretical debates discussed in Chapter 1?

Taking each of these questions in turn, it is clear that, as with lay concepts of health and illness more generally, people's views about modern medicine and the nature of their experiences of medical care and technology are complex, subtle and sophisticated. On the one hand, certain aspects of medical care and technology such as medicines and drugs, the doctor–patient relationship and the nature and quality of information in the medical encounter, appear to give rise to considerable criticism. Indeed, as Britten suggests, medicines and drugs are powerful metonyms for "the doctor". As such, criticism of one may imply criticism of the other. Certainly there appears to be evidence of a strong "anti-drugs" culture among certain segments of the lay populace, although views seem to differ according to the particular drugs in question. Moreover, the growing popularity of "complementary" therapies may, at least in part, be due to the "failures" of biomedicine and the appeal to more "holistic", "patient-centred" forms of healing, coupled with the use of non-invasive, "natural" treatments.

On the other hand, however, it is equally clear that the lay populace still place considerable faith in doctors, and continue to look to medicine for a "solution" to their ills. In particular, the evidence presented in this volume seems to suggest that, although not devoid of criticism, high-technology medicine tends to be greeted with a considerable degree of reverence and respect by the lay populace. Indeed, as Sharma suggests, even the growth of complementary therapies does not imply a wholesale rejection of orthodox medicine. Rather, patterns of dual usage remain very much the "norm" and there is little evidence to suggest that the lay populace are turning their backs on modern medicine.

Although this lay ambivalence may be rooted in traditional beliefs and commonsense knowledge, coupled with an increasing "disenchantment" with scientific rationality, it is equally clear that the media play a critical role in the framing and shaping of lay experience, including views on modern medicine – what Giddens (1991) refers to as the "mediation of experience" in "late" modernity. Indeed, in adopting this "mediatory" stance, one that plays up the "successes" as well as the "failures" of modern medicine, the media not only contributes to, but feeds off, this lay ambivalence in a mutually reinforcing way.

These issues become even more complicated in the light of the evidence presented here, which suggests that lay views on the merits of modern medicine are likely to differ according to whether it is being considered in general or personal terms. Indeed, when viewed "at a distance" there appears to be considerably more room for scepticism. In contrast, when considered in the context of personal or family illness, the picture is likely to be very different. In addition, as Britten's chapter suggests, lay views are likely to differ according to whether "orthodox" or "unorthodox" accounts are being given. In this respect, a key question concerns the extent to which people consistently hold just one view (i.e. "orthodox" *or* "unorthodox"), or draw upon both according to the social context. Certainly Cornwell's (1984) discussion of "public" and "private" accounts of health and illness suggests the latter interpretation. Moreover, the extent to which "unorthodox" accounts are allowed to surface in the medical encounter may also have a crucial bearing upon levels of "compliance" and patient "satisfaction" with medical care.

As Bendelow's chapter in particular suggests, this ambivalence is thrown into critical relief in the context of chronic pain and illness. On the one hand, the long-term nature of the illness and medicine's limited ability to help means that this is a context fraught with potential conflict as lay and medical worlds "clash" and patients become the real "experts" in managing their conditions. On the other hand, the nature of chronic illness, particularly life-threatening conditions, means that, despite its limitations, modern medicine is frequently their "best hope". Indeed, as other chapters in this volume suggest, the chronically sick and disabled, and those on long-term treatment regimens, may in fact be the least critical of modern medicine – something that, in part at least, is confounded by age. Moreover, as Gerhardt suggests, the relationship of the chronically ill to modern medicine is caught up in a whole range of moral issues and ethical dilemmas in which they have to "prove" themselves "worthy" of treatment. Indeed, even on the hotly contested terrain of human reproduction, there is evidence to suggest that women may in fact want *more* rather than less medical technology, and that this is experienced as liberating rather than oppressive (see Chs 9 and 10).

In short, it is in contexts such as these that the janus face of modern medicine is most evident, being at one and the same time a fountain of hope and font of despair; an "illegitimate reification" and a "fixed point of reference on a terrain of uncertainty"; a source of "oppression" and a means of "liberation". Certainly, in their stress on the rational actor, sociologists in the past may have neglected these seemingly "contradictory" features of lay thought. However, this does not mean that lay thought is "irrational". Rather, it possesses a logic and wisdom of its own and people appear to operate quite happily with "dual ideologies" without too much "cognitive dissonance".

Turning to the second main question, as Radley suggests, the lay evaluation of modern medicine is complicated by the fact that it touches our biographies as much as it enters our bodies. As such, in the highly charged context of health and illness, it is experienced and understood in far more intimate and personal terms than other services and products. Nevertheless, beyond these personal shades of meaning, it is possible to identify a number of key criteria that serve to structure the lay evaluation of modern medicine. In this respect, as we have seen, key aspects of medical technology include its "life-saving" nature, its "quality of life" enhancing capacities, its "iatrogenic" consequences, and the degree to which it is viewed as "unethical" or "unnatural". Certainly, as various chapters in this volume suggest, the "natural–unnatural" dichotomy tends to be a recurrent feature of lay thought. Yet as Britten rightly suggests, lay perceptions of what is "natural" and "unnatural" are far from obvious. As such, they clearly warrant further empirical investigation. In addition, particularly in today's health service, the degree to which medical treatment is perceived to be "effective" and "good value for money" also comes to the fore for politicians, managers and the public alike.

Underpinning all these criteria, of course, lies the public perception and lay evaluation of risk. Indeed, as shall be discussed below, risk becomes a key existential parameter of life in late modernity; an issue that is as pertinent to the medical arena as it is to the broader social and industrial landscape. Yet as Gabe and Bury rightly argue, these claims need to be tempered by further empirical investigation as to how far this is actually experienced and what impact social contexts (including structural factors such as age, class, gender and ethnicity) have upon the lay perception and management of risk in daily life.

What, then are the factors that shape the lay evaluation of modern medicine? Building on a previous conceptual framework developed by Calnan (1988), it is possible to identify at least six key factors at both the macro and micro-levels, which are likely to influence the lay evaluation of modern medicine and medical care. First, at the broadest level, we suggest that the socio-political values, including professional ideologies, upon which the health care system is based will structure, in a very general way, what lay people expect. In particular, the different values and professional ideologies of state-run and market-based systems of health care are likely to influence what patients themselves come to expect in the medical marketplace. Thus, although phrases such as "don't waste the doctor's time with trivia" or "only use the hospital accident and emergency department for 'emergencies'" are common examples of the philosophy of service providers in the National Health Service – values that, to some extent, appear to have been taken on board by patients themselves – it is doubtful whether such findings would be replicated in the context of privately financed health care where both supply and doctor's income are meant to respond to patient demands. In truth of course, both these models are ideal types, and it is clear that the National Health Service is currently moving or being pushed towards a form of mixed-economy health care in which the division between consumerism and paternalistic rationality is becoming blurred.

Remaining at the macro-level, it is also clear that, as mentioned above, the media play a powerful role not only in the shaping of lay views and evaluations of modern medicine, but also in the profiling of risks in contemporary society. In this respect, as we have seen, the media may play both a "mystificatory" and a "demystificatory" role, highlighting not only the positive aspects of modern medicine such as hip replacements and organ transplants, but also the "atrocity tales" such as tranquillizer dependence. In addition, media influences may also occur in other less direct ways, including the shaping of lay beliefs about health and illness and the "re-skilling" of the lay populace through the provision of information (see below). In this sense, the media may be both "creators" and "conveyors" of lay views concerning a wide range of medical and social issues, located as they are at the critical juncture between social and scientific rationality. This in turn, leads us to the third key factor in our conceptual model.

As various chapters suggest, lay concepts and images of health and illness are likely to have a crucial bearing upon people's judgements about medicine and health care. Put simply, lay concepts of health and illness will structure people's ideas about what constitutes health care and their evaluations of it. Although it is difficult to pinpoint precisely the most significant sources of influence on lay images of health and illness, they are probably a product of a complex intermixing of personal biography, socio-cultural beliefs and circumstances, and professional ideologies. Thus those with low health norms, such as the disadvantaged, may see health largely in terms of the absence of disease and are likely to define health care primarily in terms of the provision of curative services. In contrast, those with more "positive" elements in their concepts of health and illness such as the inclusion of mental and physical wellbeing, are more likely to define health care in terms of the provision of services for curative and preventive care (such as health screening or well-women clinics). Consequently, they will evaluate health care within this alternative frame of reference.

The fourth element in the model is closely tied to the third in that lay concepts of health and illness are also likely to influence the reasons *why* an individual seeks medical help in each specific instance, as well as their perceptions of health problems and their responses to them. In other words, although the concept of patient expectations has been shown to be largely redundant, lay evaluation can be understood more simply in terms of the specific reasons why the sufferers and their families sought medical care in each specific instance (i.e. their "goals"). Thus, to take just one example, patients may seek health care, particularly from a general practitioner, for a wide variety of complaints. In each particular instance they will have specific needs and make specific demands that they believe should be met by those providing the service. In this context, the family doctor may have to play a variety of different roles that include the doctor as "technician" to treat minor cuts and bruises, the doctor as "diagnostician" and information giver for problematic signs and symptoms, the doctor as "advice giver" and reassurer for anxious parents and the doctor as "counsellor" for psychosocial problems. In each of this short list of examples, patients will make different demands upon the doctor and will evaluate medical care according to whether or not those demands are met. Certainly, as Britten's chapter shows, patients are often critical if their GP simply reaches for the prescription pad.

Again closely allied to this fourth factor, the fifth element in the model suggests that the nature of the individual's (and close social network's) past experiences will also have a crucial bearing upon their evaluations of medical care. The uncertainties and unpredictabilities that surround illness and the professional medical care provided to manage and treat it suggest that patients may only become knowledgeable when they or their network of friends and relations actually experience medical care. Thus, any expectations they may have will be created and influenced by their subsequent experience. Clearly, as discussed above, these issues are crucial in the context of chronic illness where the accumulation of past experiences of "success" and "failure" in relation to modern medicine, and the growing sense of "expertise" on the part of patients themselves, may lead to a mixture of hope and despair. In addition, it is also clear that previous use and experience of complementary therapies may lead to a more critical attitude towards orthodox medicine.

Finally, the sixth factor in the model, and one that underpins many of the issues discussed above, concerns the influence of socio-demographic factors. These it is suggested, should be included as *mediatory* elements in the model as they are likely to have an influence upon each of the other factors considered above. For example, as we have seen, factors such as age, gender, class, ethnicity and health status are all, in their differing ways, likely to influence the lay evaluation of medical care. Certainly one of the strongest and most consistent findings here concerns the way in which the lay evaluation of modern medicine and medical care appears to vary according to age. As suggested, this might be explained by different health problems and experiences of medical care associated with ageing. Alternatively, it may be related to different "norms" about health associated with different age groups. Finally, it may be related to ideological differences in the approach to medical care associated with different generations – or a mixture of all these factors.

These then are the six key elements that, building on and extending Calnan's (1988) previous model and the evidence presented here, are believed to shape the lay evaluation of modern medicine and medical care. Clearly, however, this is a tentative model, and further research is needed in order to test its applicability across a variety of health care settings and differing social groups.

Finally, in turning to the last question, what does all this tell us about the relationship between modern medicine and the lay populace in the contemporary era, and what light does it shed upon some of the more macro-focused theoretical debates discussed in Chapter 1?

Clearly, on the basis of the evidence presented here, the notion of a "blanket dependence" on modern medicine or the fabrication of "docile bodies" appears to have a somewhat hollow ring to it, resulting in a largely "overdrawn" view of medical power, dominance and control. In this respect, the lay public are not simply passive and dependent upon modern medicine, nor are they necessarily duped by medical ideology and technology. Indeed, as Cornwell's (1984) framework suggests, rationalizing processes may not be carried through everywhere in all social groups at the same pace and at the same time. As such, the "rate" of medicalization depends upon the state of readiness of different sub-cultures, and individuals within these sub-cultural groups, to allow it to take place.

Certainly there is evidence to suggest that a "critical distance" is beginning to open up between modern medicine and the lay populace and that people are becoming more "ambivalent" and sceptical; a trend that, in turn, is linked to a broader set of changes that is sweeping through contemporary western societies. As Giddens (1990, 1991) suggests, we are entering a period of "high" or "late" modernity – a "post-traditional" social order (Giddens 1994) – in which the consequences of modernity are becoming ever more radicalized and universalized. Within this context, "active" forms of trust and "radical" forms of doubt become a pervasive feature of modern critical reasoning; one that modernity institutionalizes by insisting that all knowledge is tentative, corrigible and therefore open to subsequent revision or abandonment (Giddens 1991). Here, systems of accumulated expertise come to represent multiple sources of authority that are frequently contested and divergent in their implications. It is in this sense that late modernity displays a high degree of institutional *reflexivity*, involving the routine incorporation of new knowledge and information into environments of action, which are thereby reconstituted or reorganized in the process (Giddens 1991). In short, modernity becomes its own theme (Beck 1992).

As a consequence of these processes, the relationship between modern medicine and the lay populace becomes increasingly built around a reflexively organized dialectic of trust and doubt. Indeed, while the nature of modern social life is deeply bound up with mechanisms of trust in abstract systems, this is nonetheless a very special sort of trust; namely an "active" form of trust that, as the name implies, has to be continually "won" and retained in the face of growing doubt and uncertainty (Giddens 1994). In short, as Giddens notes, many different relationships between lay experience and abstract systems exist within late modernity:

> Attitudes of trust, as well as more pragmatic acceptance, scepticism, rejection and withdrawal, uneasily co-exist in the social space linking individual activities and expert systems. Lay attitudes towards science, technology and other esoteric forms of expertise, in the age of high modernity, express the same mixture of attitudes of reverence and reserve, approval and disquiet, enthusiasm and antipathy, which philosophers and social analysts (themselves experts of a sort) express in their writings (Giddens 1991: 7).

Given these developments, risk becomes a critical issue. Indeed, in terms of the present discussion, its significance lies in the fact that widespread lay knowledge of modern risk environments serves to expose the "limits" of so-called "expertise", thus serving to weaken or further undermine people's faith and confidence in official pronouncements, including those of the medical establishment, concerning public safety and danger. Clearly, as suggested earlier, the media play a crucial role in these processes and the broader "demystification" of science and technology.

It is in this context that notions of lay "re-skilling" (i.e. the re-acquisition or re-appropriation of knowledge and skills) and the emergence of "life political agenda" come to the fore as pervasive reactions to the expropriating effects of modern abstract systems of knowledge and expertise:

> . . . technical knowledge is continually re-appropriated by lay agents as part of their routine dealings with abstract systems . . . Modern life is a complex affair and there are many "filter-back" processes whereby technical knowledge, in one shape or another, is re-appropriated by lay persons and routinely applied in the course of their day-to-day activities . . . Processes of re-appropriation relate to all aspects of social life – for example medical treatments, child rearing, or sexual pleasure (Giddens 1991: 144–6).

On the one hand, the nature of lay re-skilling suggests that individuals are increasingly coming to "take back" control over matters of health and illness, and returning to "natural" rather than "technological" forms of health and healing in an attempt to "de-medicalize" society. Certainly, the extent of "non-compliance" with medical treatment and advice and the growing popularity of "complementary therapies" appear to support such an interpretation. Similarly, on a more collective scale, the growth of self-help groups (Kelleher 1994), environmental health movements (Williams and Popay 1994), and other developments such as the upsurge of anti-vivisectionist activity (Elston 1994), are particularly good examples of the growth of "life political agenda's" in late modernity. On the other hand, the notion of lay re-skilling may also suggest that, far from rejecting modern medical technology, individuals are increasingly coming to "reappropriate" it for their own rather than professional ends as a potential means of "liberation". Indeed, as we have seen, one of the key themes to emerge from this volume, particularly in the context of women's lives, has been the extent to which medical technology may actually be seen as a "resource" rather than a means of social "oppression" in controlling the "natural", "sick" or "recalcitrant" body.

In summary, as we have suggested, lay "ambivalence" towards modern medicine may fruitfully be located within the broader contours and existential parameters of life in late modernity; a reflexive social order in which active forms of trust intersect with radical forms of doubt in a dialectical interplay, and processes of "lay re-skilling" and the emergence of "life political agenda" come to the fore as a response to the expropriating effects of modern abstract systems. Clearly, issues of class and social structure mesh closely with these arguments and further empirical specification is required as to the precise extent and pervasiveness of these processes within different segments of the lay populace (see Ch. 4 on this point). At a broader level, these developments pose significant new questions concerning the "fate" of medical power and professional dominance in the late modern age; issues that, in turn, extend and develop the *deprofessionalization* (Haug 1973, 1988) and *proletarianization* (McKinlay & Arches 1985) theses discussed in Chapter 1. Taken together, these developments, at the very least, suggest that a critical reconfiguration of professional power and dominance is beginning to take place in contemporary western society.

In conclusion, in this world of uncertain times, one thing remains clear: namely, that lay people are not simply passive or active, dependent or independent, believers or sceptics. Rather, they are a complex mixture of all these things (and much more besides). Without wishing to sound too postmodern, social reality, in truth, is both complex and contradictory, and we would do well to remember this as we edge ever closer towards the twenty-first century.

References

Beck, U. 1992. *Risk society: towards a new modernity*. London: Sage.

Calnan, M. 1988. Towards a conceptual framework of lay evaluation of health care. *Social Science and Medicine* **27**(9), 927–33.

Cornwell, J. 1984. *Hard-earned lives: accounts of health and illness from East London*. London: Tavistock.

Elston, M. A. 1994. The anti-vivisection movement and the science of medicine. In *Challenging medicine*, J. Gabe, D. Kelleher, G. Williams (eds), 160–80. London: Routledge.

Giddens, A. 1990. *The consequences of modernity*. Cambridge: Polity.

Giddens, A. 1991. *Modernity and self-identity: self and society in the late modern age*. Cambridge: Polity.

Giddens, A. 1994. *Beyond left and right*. Cambridge: Polity.

Haug, M. 1973. Deprofessionalization: an alternative hypothesis for the future. *Sociological Review Monograph* **20**, 195–211.

Haug, M. 1988. A re-examination of the hypothesis of physician deprofessionalization. *Milbank Memorial Fund Quarterly* **66** (Supplement 2), 48–56.

Kelleher, D. 1994. Self-help groups and their relationship to medicine. In *Challenging medicine*, J. Gabe, D. Kelleher, G. Williams (eds), 104–17. London: Routledge.

McKinlay, J. & J. Arches 1985. Towards the proletarianization of physicians. *International Journal of Health Services*, **15**, 161–95.

Williams, G. & J. Popay 1994. Lay knowledge and the privilege of experience. In *Challenging medicine*, Gabe J., D. Kelleher, G. H. Williams (eds), 118–39. London: Routledge.

Index